Weight loss secrets you need to know

Why your brain, body physiology, emotions, and primordial drives want you fat and what you can do about it

By David R. Seaman, DC, MS
Author of *The DeFlame Diet*

www.deflame.com

Shadow Panther Press

Wilmington, NC

Disclaimer

This book is intended as an educational volume only; not as a medical or treatment manual. The information contained herein is not intended to take the place of professional medical care; it is not to be used for diagnosing or treating disease; it is not intended to dictate what constitutes reasonable, appropriate or best care for any given health issue; nor is it intended to be used as a substitute for any treatment that may have been prescribed by your doctor. If you have questions regarding a medical condition, always seek the advice of your physician or other qualified health professional.

The reader assumes all responsibility and risk for the use of the information in this book. Under no circumstances shall the author be held liable for any damage resulting directly or indirectly from the information contained herein.

Reference to any products, services, internet links to third parties or other information by trade name, trademark, suppliers, or otherwise does not constitute or imply its endorsement, sponsorship, or recommendation by the author.

Edited by: Tom Seaman, Shadow Panther Press
Author of Diagnosis Dystonia: Navigating the Journey

Cover design by: Kate Cozzie: www.katecozziegraphicarts.com
Photographs of lean Tom by Terry D Sandman Photography - drtsandman@aol.com

ISBN: 1720995761
ISBN-13: 978-1720995760

Table of Contents

About the Author

Dr. David Seaman wrote the first scientific article about dietary induction of chronic inflammation which has become a very important area in the emerging field of integrative medicine. His articles about pain, inflammation, diet, and obesity have been referenced by researchers at Harvard Medical School and many other universities in the United States, Canada, Brazil, Europe, Middle East, India, Australia, Russia and other Asian countries.

In 2016, Dr. Seaman wrote *The DeFlame Diet*, a layman's book that outlines the many aspects of diet-induced inflammation. *Weight Loss Secrets You Need to Know* is his second book in the DeFlame series of books. The next book to hopefully be completed by the end of 2018 is *The DeFlame Diet for Female Health*.

His DeFlame nutrition information can be found at DeFlame.com, where you can also link to his YouTube channel and Facebook page.

Dr. Seaman has been a faculty member at Palmer College of Chiropractic Florida and at National University of Health Sciences. He currently teaches nutrition for Logan College of Chiropractic.

Introduction

Weight loss and proper weight maintenance are not really about food itself. They are about our mental relationship to food, exerting control over our emotions and our body physiology, and understanding the primordial drives (survival instincts) that make us overeat. If we have a defective mental relationship with food, do not understand our emotions and body physiology in relation to body weight maintenance, and let the primordial drives run amok, odds are very strong that we will be overweight or obese. Let me give you an example…

In 2001, my brother Tom (on the cover of this book) was an active, athletic 30-year old man. He is 6'2" tall and weighed 190 pounds. He rapidly developed a chronic neurological movement disorder called cervical dystonia (a.k.a. spasmodic torticollis) and became severely disabled and unable to work. A little over 5 years later he weighed 340 pounds. He got there because his world totally changed overnight… he was in constant severe pain, mentally depressed, anxiety ridden, and felt hopeless and helpless.

He did not go to sleep until 4-5 in the morning and during the hours before bed he would snack on chips, dips, deli sandwiches, fried foods, cheese, and bread, and then wash it all down with several beers. For meals he would eat large amounts of pasta, breaded Chinese food, fried fish or chicken, fast food burgers and fries, and sometimes an entire fully loaded frozen pizza that he often covered with hot dogs and more cheese. He was living in a mindless autopilot state when it came to food, which is very common and happens to people with far less dramatic life events than Tom's.

In 2007, he forced upon himself a new mindset. Within 1 year, he lost 150 pounds and weighed 190 pounds and has kept that weight off to the present day. AND he lost the weight and has maintained his weight loss since 2007 with minimal exercise due to the limitations of his cervical (neck) dystonia...*his success was mental*. He developed and maintained a proper body weight mindset, which allowed him to control his mental relationship to food, body physiology, and the primordial eating drives. Below are pictures that illustrate his transformation, which are also on the cover of this book.

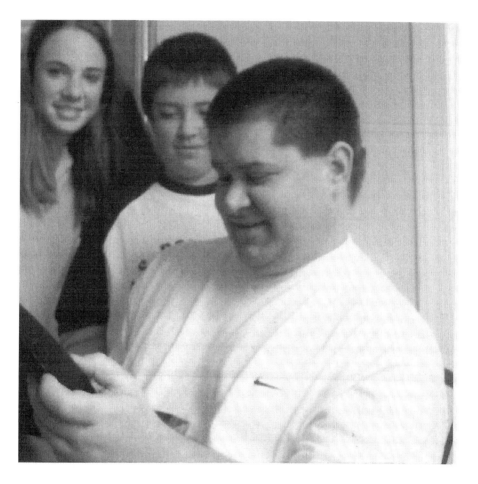

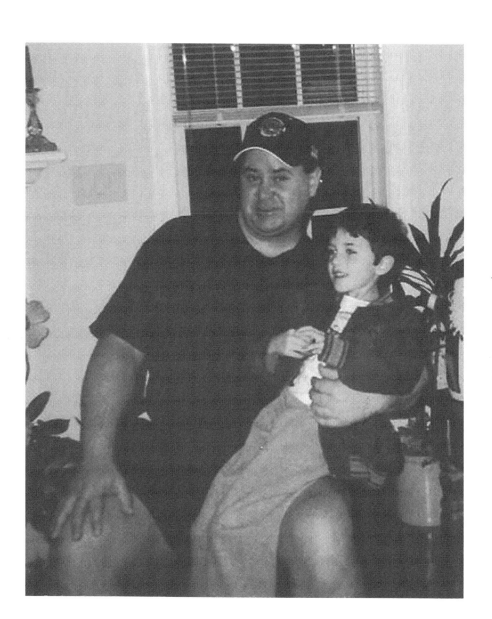

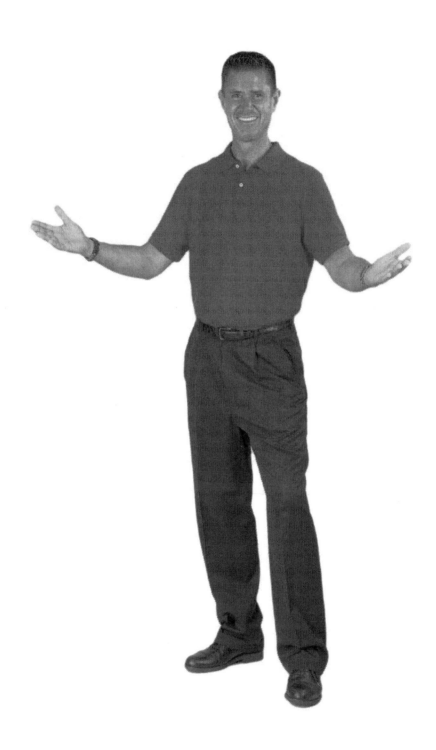

The point of *Weight Loss Secrets You Need to Know* is learning how to develop the proper mindset for engaging the weight-gain environment, which can be likened to a battlefield in which we all live. The mindset that I am referring to is self-discipline, or mindfulness if you like, which can be applied to all aspects of our lives. However, mindfulness is not the only important ingredient for proper weight management. We also need to understand our emotional relationship to food and how body physiology and primordial eating drives facilitate weight gain, and appreciate further how the power of each of these is enhanced because we now live in an obesogenic environment, which is described in upcoming chapters. If you do not understand this information, it is much more difficult to manage weight effectively.

If you would like to learn more about Tom's journey, as well as many practical skills and strategies for successfully living with *any* chronic health condition, you can read his book, *Diagnosis Dystonia: Navigating the Journey*. He is also a certified professional life coach and can help you with weight management. You can learn more about his coaching practice and order his book at www.tomseamancoaching.com.

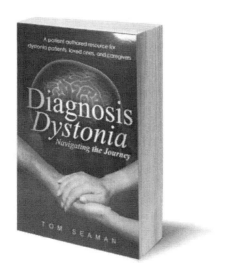

Chapter 1
The DeFlame Diet – a quick review

The DeFlame Diet was the first in a series of DeFlame books to be published – this weight loss secrets book is the second to be published. Table 1 has been reproduced from the *The DeFlame Diet* book. The foods that create a pro-inflammatory state are the same ones that make us fat and keep us fat, so they must be avoided. I refer to these pro-inflammatory foods as "dietary crack,"and this is because they generate addiction chemistry in our brains that is similar to cocaine, which makes us dietary "crackheads." The outcome is that we overeat them in quantities that are too great, such that the excess calories are stored as body fat.

Table 1. Pro-inflammatory vs DeFlame Diet vs DeFlame Ketogenic Diet

Pro-inflammatory calories	DeFlame Diet	DeFlame Ketogenic Diet
Refined sugar	Grass-fed meat and wild game	Grass-fed meat and wild game
Refined grains	Meats	Meats
Grain flour products	Wild caught fish	Wild caught fish
Trans fats	Shellfish	Shellfish
Omega-6 seed oils (corn, safflower, sunflower, peanut, etc.)	Chicken	Chicken
	Omega-3 eggs	Omega-3 eggs
	Cheese	Cheese
	Vegetables	Vegetables
	Salads (leafy vegetables)	Salads (leafy vegetables)
	Fruit	*No fruit*
	Roots/tubers (potato, yams, sweet potato)	*No roots/tubers*
	Nuts (raw or dry roasted)	Nuts (raw or dry roasted)
	Omega-3 seeds: hemp, chia, flax seeds	Omega-3 seeds: hemp, chia, flax seeds
	Dark chocolate	*Sugar free dark chocolate*
	Spices of all kinds	Spices of all kinds
	Olive oil, coconut oil,	Olive oil, coconut oil,

	butter, cream, avocado, bacon	butter, cream, avocado, bacon
	Red wine and dark beer	Red wine
	Coffee and tea (green tea is best option)	Coffee and tea (green tea is best option)
		No legumes and whole grains

Be aware that even the calorie-rich foods that create a DeFlamed state can make you fat and keep you fat, so they must be eaten in amounts that meet individual caloric needs. In other words, anyone who consumes an excess of calories from cheese, potatoes, nuts, seeds, dark chocolate, oils, butter, avocado, and bacon, will gain weight and become obese. In contrast, no one can become obese by only eating vegetables and this is because no one can eat the volume of vegetables needed to create a caloric excess that promotes the accumulation of body fat. This means that most of us need to dramatically increase our intake of vegetables and be careful to not overeat the calorie-rich foods that are included in *The DeFlame Diet*. By doing this and simultaneously avoiding "dietary crack," it is virtually impossible to become overweight or obese.

Notice that Table 1 also presents The DeFlame Ketogenic Diet. Many people do well on a ketogenic diet, which has now become very popular for weight loss, health promotion, and inflammation reduction. A ketogenic diet contains less than 50 grams of carbohydrate per day. This means no sugar and flour at all, and in most cases, no grains, beans, roots/tubers, and fruit. Fat calories are the primary focus. This style of eating works for some people but not for others. My view is to choose foods that suit your mind and body, and allow you to achieve and maintain normal markers of inflammation as outlined in Chapter 9 of *The DeFlame Diet* book. I discuss the ketogenic diet in more detail in Chapter 33 in the *The DeFlame Diet*.

As described in *The DeFlame Diet* book, the obesity state is associated with chronic inflammation. If you have read the *The*

DeFlame Diet, you will recall that our adipose tissue mass (body fat) is anti-inflammatory when we are lean; however, as body fat accumulates, the immune cell profile changes to one that is pro-inflammatory. The outcome is that obese body fat immune cells behave as if there is a low-grade infection or autoimmune disease.

If you have not yet read *The DeFlame Diet* book, you should. Here is why…

- Diet and nutrition has become such a complicated and confusing area that we need a grounded view on nutrition. What I mean is, we need to think in simple terms. Will this food "inflame" me or "DeFlame" me? That is the question to ask before putting food in our mouths.

- The reason for thinking in "inflame vs DeFlame" terms is because all diseases are actually chronic inflammatory states. Benign conditions like chronic aches and pains, osteoarthritis, malaise, and depression are all pro-inflammatory states. Most people spend half of their lives suffering with these benign conditions before succumbing to a more lethal pro-inflammatory state, such as heart disease, cancer, or Alzheimer's disease. Even the aging process is a chronic inflammatory state, which has been termed inflammaging. So, we want to anti-inflammage versus pro-inflammage.

- *The DeFlame Diet* outlines the nature of chronic inflammation, how we become inflamed, how to track inflammation, and how to reduce chronic inflammation throughout our lifespan.

You can order a hard copy and Kindle version of *The DeFlame Diet* book on Amazon.com.

Volume discounts for hard copies of *The DeFlame Diet* and *Weight Loss Secrets You Need to Know* are available at DeFlame.com.

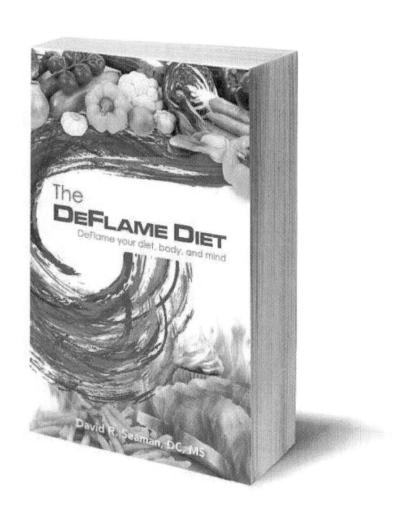

Chapter 2
Eating and the pursuit of happiness –
The fat person's attitude that needs to change

The pursuit of happiness is a problematic notion for modern man, which will become obvious to you by the time you finish this chapter. Happiness is really about chronic pleasure-seeking, and when this involves high-calorie foods, obesity is the unavoidable outcome. Please read this chapter carefully.

Perhaps the most famous use of the word "happiness" is found in the Declaration of Independence, wherein Thomas Jefferson wrote that "we are endowed by the Creator with certain unalienable rights, that among these are life, liberty, and the pursuit of happiness."

Not well known is that Jefferson's thinking was influenced by John Locke, a famous English philosopher. Locke died in 1704, long before the Declaration of Independence was written. Locke stated that Nature's law and reason indicates that we are all equal and independent and that, "no one ought to harm another in his life, health, liberty, or possessions." Classical liberal philosophy, which bears little resemblance to the ideologies expressed in the current liberal-conservative vortex, further interprets this to also mean that private property is a natural right, which all individuals have. In other words, as you will see, it would have been better for Jefferson to not have suggested that we pursue happiness and instead stated that, "we are endowed by the Creator with certain unalienable rights, that among these are life, liberty, and the ownership of property."

The notion that we should pursue happiness is advanced in movies, books, television shows, and by family, friends, and loved ones, and no one gives it a second thought or remotely comprehends the trouble it causes. Pursuing happiness is a great slogan for selling products and justifying foolish behaviors. For example, I have heard people say numerous times that eating French fries and desserts makes them happy, so why should they stop? The answer is simple: Because eating a high-calorie pro-inflammatory diet will eventually lead you to a most brutal pit of misery, as in the future development of severe chronic pain, breast cancer, prostate cancer, diabetes, vascular diseases, or some other awful debilitating disease that will destroy your life and can wreak substantial mental havoc and financial collateral damage upon you and your loved ones. Clearly, regular dietary "hits" of "happiness" ultimately lead to substantial unhappiness and this happens sooner rather than later for most people as life flies by, particularly as we get older.

The problem with "happiness" is that most people do not understand its physiologic nature. From the perspective of body physiology, happiness is a transient state of elevated physiology expressed as increased pleasure chemicals, such as dopamine, which means it is biologically similar to the response one gets from any addictive substance. In other words, happiness is actually about constant pleasure seeking and overstimulation of the senses.

Unfortunately, little thought is actually given when friends and loved ones wish "happiness" upon each other. The likely reason people do this is because the human mind inherently thinks in terms of extremes when it comes to many topics, including happiness; that is, we think we can only be happy or unhappy. From a psychophysiologic perspective, this is a preposterous notion, and no one should be allowed to grow up thinking in this manner.

The psychophysiologic goal ideally is to "not be unhappy," and this is not a trivial semantic issue at all. It is discussed in religions, by poets and philosophers, and by psychologists:

> In the Bhagavad Gita we are urged to pursue a
> state of, "evenness in pleasure and pain," each of

which happens to all of us as a matter of being alive. From a behavioral perspective, The Gita further urges us to control our exposure to external sensory stimuli that create transient desire/pleasure surges and the subsequent opposite effect...the feeling of loss and the need for constant sense-derived pleasure, which we interpret as "happiness."

The Four Noble Truths of Buddhism deliver a similar message as The Gita. The message is that "life is suffering." And when we know this and truly understand it, we will not be unhappy and not care about being happy. Buddhist philosophy outlines how to properly negotiate suffering and it is referred to as the Noble Eightfold Path, which includes right understanding, thought, speech, action, livelihood, effort, mindfulness, and concentration.

Many sections of the Bible deliver this message as well, especially in the context of the dangers associated with temptation and excessive pleasure seeking.

From Rudyard Kipling's poem "If," he states: "If you can meet with triumph (happiness) and disaster (unhappiness) and treat those two imposters just the same..." In other words, we should be indifferent to the ups and downs in life and pursue a state of emotional evenness, which means "not being unhappy."

In Dr. M Scott Peck's famous book, *The Road Less Travelled*, he describes that life is difficult, and we must deal with our problems by engaging in our lives, which makes one's life less difficult, more focused and productive, and *not unhappy.*

Clearly, the notion that one should pursue happiness is spiritually, psychologically, and physiologically absurd. More recently on this scene is Dr. Jordan Peterson, a Canadian psychologist, who outlines why life is difficult and filled with suffering, and how to combat being plummeted into the depths of nihilism and misery by pursuing a life of meaning. Peterson discusses this topic in his YouTube videos and his book, *12 Rules for Life: An antidote to chaos.*

In short, when one's life has meaning and purpose, there is no reason to pursue transient surges of happiness that are derived from unhealthy external stimuli. Feelings of happiness occur naturally at various times when we pursue worthy goals. Otherwise, our base emotional state should be one of evenness that I call, "not being unhappy."

When we consider that being a living human is difficult in its own right, and then further compromised by trials, tribulations, losses, pain, suffering, sickness, disease, and eventually death, it is actually surprising that life is not only a thoroughly unhappy state all the time. And perhaps, this is why happiness is visualized to be such a desirable goal, because people desperately want relief from the pit of misery that is their lives to varying degrees. To the point of this book, the repeated consumption of dietary crack is one way that people get a transient dopamine surge of pleasure/happiness that temporarily removes one from the pit of misery. It is important to understand that this behavioral activity of pleasure engagement from dietary crack was not historically available to us.

Until the modern day, eating was habitual (we have been doing it since before we even consciously knew that we existed) and primordial (without food we would die), but it was NOT about pleasure. Eating was not about pleasure because breads, sweetened cereals, fast-foods, and dessert-type foods, which you should think of as "dietary crack," did not exist when we were hunting and gathering; save for the occasional bees' nest full of honey. The closest we had historically to a sweetened food would be fruit.

Today, eating is about pleasure at a substantial hedonistic level, meaning that eating is a sensually self-indulgent activity for most people at all levels of the economic spectrum and pursued throughout the day. And when one gets the "taste" and pleasure "hit" from dietary crack at an early age, then just like addictive drugs, dietary crack consumption becomes a goal because it neurologically equates to pleasure and happiness. The next time you are in a restaurant, watch how people have a drug-like response when they taste dietary crack – they get a dopamine pleasure response, which equates to a momentary state of "happiness."

A better goal than "happiness" – not being unhappy

We basically have three mental states that we shift in and out of, those being unhappiness, not being unhappy (at peace), and happiness. Unhappiness is associated with most negative emotions, such as anger, hostility, frustration, helplessness, hopelessness, depression, and anxiety, which correlate with too much inflammation in the body. These unhappiness feelings can be useful in the short term to help us make course correcting decisions to improve our lives and move out of the domain of unhappiness. In other words, we should embrace transient states of unhappiness to learn about making better life decisions to become "not unhappy."

Depression is one of the most common negative mental states in which one can live – it is a chronic state of unhappiness and increased inflammation. Any legitimately depressed person will tell you that they would just like to "not be unhappy" and feel normal again. They are not looking for a rush of pleasure to create a moment of fun and "happiness" – they want to be "not unhappy."

In contrast with a depressed person, the average individual lives mostly in a state of "not being unhappy" but strives for constant surges of happiness, and from what I can tell, this is largely due the endless stream of advertising propaganda that is delivered to us 24 hours a day. Not well known is that modern advertising to consumers began after World War I. Here is a brief history for perspective.

President Woodrow Wilson invited Edward Bernays, a prominent propagandist and the nephew of Sigmund Freud, to be part of the US group that went to France for the signing of the Treaty of Versailles, because of his participation in Wilson's Committee on Public Information. The CPI, as it was referred, was responsible for getting Americans to shift their sentiments from being "anti-war" to "pro-war," part of which involved the creation of the slogan promoting the notion that Americans fight for "freedom and democracy."

Upon his return from France, Bernays realized that if propaganda could be so successful for promoting war, it could be used to steer society during times of peace, which led him to start his new propaganda business in New York City, which he called Public Relations. Interestingly, Edward Bernays, known now as the Father of Public Relations, stylized his consumerist propaganda based on the work of his uncle, Sigmund Freud. Space does not permit a detailed description here of Bernays and his work – my suggestion is to read articles published in The Conversation[1] and at Smithsonian.com.[2] For a most detailed view of Bernays, watch Adam Curtis' documentary entitled *The Century of the Self*.[3] Part 1 is devoted to Bernays, wherein humans are described as "happiness machines" which need to be directed to buy products that we don't need to achieve "happiness."

The outcome of the Bernays style of propaganda to which the public has been exposed to over the past 100 years is a mental state of mind in which a normal peaceful state of "not being unhappy" is not enough and not normal. We have been conditioned to ceaselessly pursue an unsustainable emotional dopamine-related experience called happiness. This applies to all consumer products, vacationing, television watching, sporting activities, political ideologies, emotional pursuits, and in the context of this book...the mindless consumption of unhealthy, high calorie foods, which leads to pain, obesity, and chronic disease.

So, the battlefield of weight management includes dealing with our mental/emotional relationship with food, controlling our body physiology, understanding the primordial drives, AND dealing with brutal food propaganda. I will tackle food propaganda a bit more in the remainder of this chapter and then outline an action plan that will be expanded upon in the remainder of this book.

The USDA and its food propaganda over the past 100 years
In 2010, the United States Department of Agriculture (USDA) published Dietary Guidelines for Americans. The full document can be acquired if you google the title. On the following page is Table 2-2, which lists the most commonly eaten foods by Americans ages 2 and older. Notice that the primary calories consumed by all age groups are refined sugar, flour, oils, milk, meat, chicken, and cheese. No vegetables or fruit make the top 25 most commonly consumed foods in any age category...now that is "impressive" in terms of the pursuit of disease in general, and obesity in the context of this book.

TABLE 2 2. Top 25 Sources of Calories Among Americans Ages 2 Years and Older, NHANES 2005-2006[a]

Rank	Overall, Ages 2+ yrs (Mean kcal/d; Total daily calories = 2,157)	Children and Adolescents, Ages 2-18 yrs (Mean kcal/d; Total daily calories = 2,027)	Adults and Older Adults, Ages 19+ yrs (Mean kcal/d; Total daily calories = 2,199)
1	Grain-based desserts[b] (138 kcal)	Grain-based desserts (138 kcal)	Grain-based desserts (138 kcal)
2	Yeast breads[c] (129 kcal)	Pizza (136 kcal)	Yeast breads (134 kcal)
3	Chicken and chicken mixed dishes[d] (121 kcal)	Soda/energy/sports drinks (118 kcal)	Chicken and chicken mixed dishes (123 kcal)
4	Soda/energy/sports drinks[e] (114 kcal)	Yeast breads (114 kcal)	Soda/energy/sports drinks (112 kcal)
5	Pizza (98 kcal)	Chicken and chicken mixed dishes (113 kcal)	Alcoholic beverages (106 kcal)
6	Alcoholic beverages (82 kcal)	Pasta and pasta dishes (91 kcal)	Pizza (86 kcal)
7	Pasta and pasta dishes[f] (81 kcal)	Reduced fat milk (86 kcal)	Tortillas, burritos, tacos (85 kcal)
8	Tortillas, burritos, tacos[g] (80 kcal)	Dairy desserts (76 kcal)	Pasta and pasta dishes (78 kcal)
9	Beef and beef mixed dishes[h] (64 kcal)	Potato/corn/other chips (70 kcal)	Beef and beef mixed dishes (71 kcal)
10	Dairy desserts[i] (62 kcal)	Ready-to-eat cereals (65 kcal)	Dairy desserts (58 kcal)
11	Potato/corn/other chips (56 kcal)	Tortillas, burritos, tacos (63 kcal)	Burgers (53 kcal)
12	Burgers (53 kcal)	Whole milk (60 kcal)	Regular cheese (51 kcal)
13	Reduced fat milk (51 kcal)	Candy (56 kcal)	Potato/corn/other chips (51 kcal)
14	Regular cheese (49 kcal)	Fruit drinks (55 kcal)	Sausage, franks, bacon, and ribs (49 kcal)
15	Ready-to-eat cereals (49 kcal)	Burgers (55 kcal)	Nuts/seeds and nut/seed mixed dishes (47 kcal)
16	Sausage, franks, bacon, and ribs (49 kcal)	Fried white potatoes (52 kcal)	Fried white potatoes (46 kcal)
17	Fried white potatoes (48 kcal)	Sausage, franks, bacon, and ribs (47 kcal)	Ready-to-eat cereals (44 kcal)
18	Candy (47 kcal)	Regular cheese (43 kcal)	Candy (44 kcal)
19	Nuts/seeds and nut/seed mixed dishes[j] (42 kcal)	Beef and beef mixed dishes (43 kcal)	Eggs and egg mixed dishes (42 kcal)
20	Eggs and egg mixed dishes[k] (39 kcal)	100% fruit juice, not orange/grapefruit (35 kcal)	Rice and rice mixed dishes (41 kcal)
21	Rice and rice mixed dishes[l] (36 kcal)	Eggs and egg mixed dishes (30 kcal)	Reduced fat milk (39 kcal)
22	Fruit drinks[m] (36 kcal)	Pancakes, waffles, and French toast (29 kcal)	Quickbreads (36 kcal)
23	Whole milk (33 kcal)	Crackers (28 kcal)	Other fish and fish mixed dishes[n] (30 kcal)
24	Quickbreads[o] (32 kcal)	Nuts/seeds and nut/seed mixed dishes (27 kcal)	Fruit drinks (29 kcal)
25	Cold cuts (27 kcal)	Cold cuts (24 kcal)	Salad dressing (29 kcal)

Imagine for a moment that this dismal eating behavior that applies to the average American across the lifestyle spectrum is actually the outcome of 100 years of conditioning and reflects adherence to established government policies. Many might think that this is an impossible notion…well, take a look at the images on the next several pages that were produced by the USDA that span from 1912 to 1992 (Milk 1912, Corn and cottage cheese 1914-1918, Simple Suppers are Best 1919, Vitamin Donuts WWII, Ice Cream Cake 1950, Food Pyramid 1992).

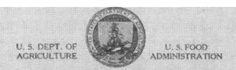

U. S. DEPT. OF
AGRICULTURE

U. S. FOOD
ADMINISTRATION

MILK

The Best Food We Have

GIVE YOUR CHILDREN MILK

A QUART a day for every child, if possible, a pint without fail. Plenty of milk will help give all your children, big and little, the chance for health they ought to have. Buy more milk and less meat and your family will be better fed.

MILK HELPS YOUR CHILDREN TO GROW. Besides well-known food substances it has something special which they must have to grow. Your children can get a little of this from other foods, but not enough. Give your boys and girls milk for their chance to grow.

MILK HELPS YOUR CHILDREN TO KEEP WELL. Look at children who do not get milk, but get tea and coffee instead. Aren't most of them pale and sickly? There are always very many sick children in cities and in countries where milk is scarce. When milk prices go up and mothers begin to economize on milk more children become sick. Do not let your children run this risk. Give them fresh, clean milk and help them to grow up strong and well and win in their fight against disease. Save on other things if you must, but not on milk, your child's best food.

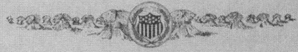

United States Food Leaflet No. 11.

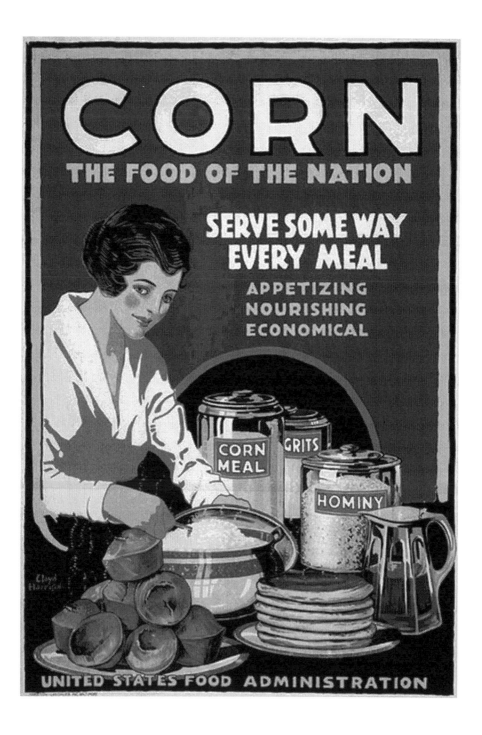

EAT MORE COTTAGE CHEESE

One pound of beef, or

One pound of pork, or

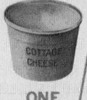

→SUPPLIES MORE PROTEIN THAN——

One pound of lamb, or

ONE POUND

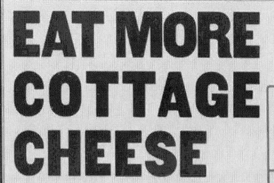

One pound of veal, or

YOU'LL NEED LESS MEAT

One pound of fowl

A Postal Card Will Bring Recipes

for using this meat substitute

U. S. DEPARTMENT OF AGRICULTURE, WASHINGTON, D. C.

COTTAGE CHEESE OR MEAT **ASK YOUR POCKETBOOK**

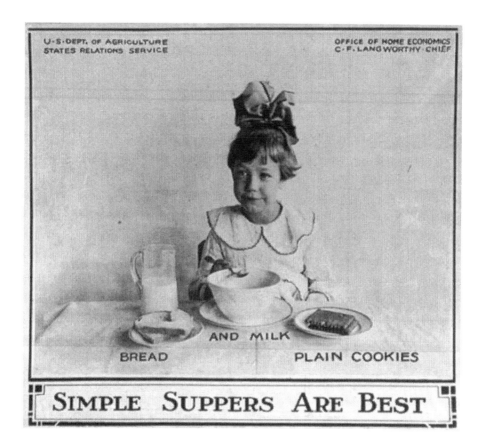

U·S·DEPT. OF AGRICULTURE
STATES RELATIONS SERVICE

OFFICE OF HOME ECONOMICS
C·F·LANGWORTHY·CHIEF

AND MILK

BREAD

PLAIN COOKIES

SIMPLE SUPPERS ARE BEST

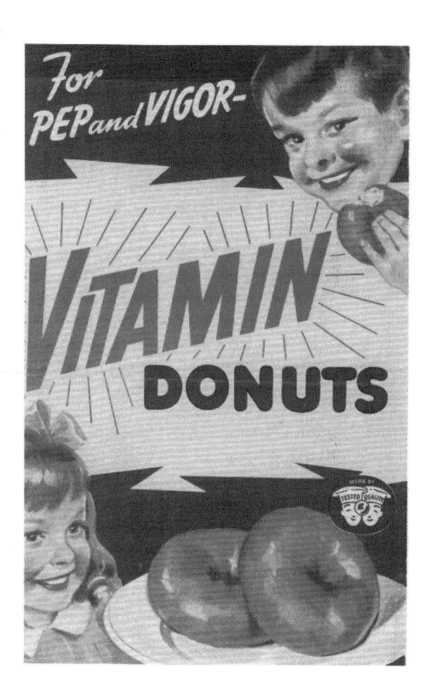

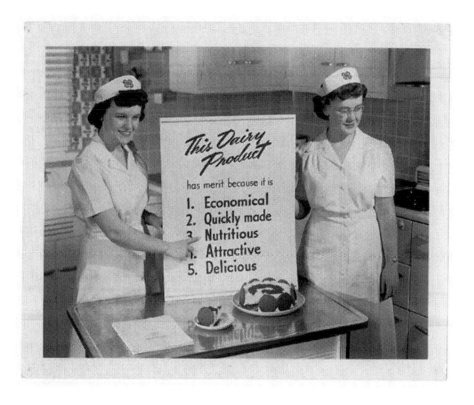

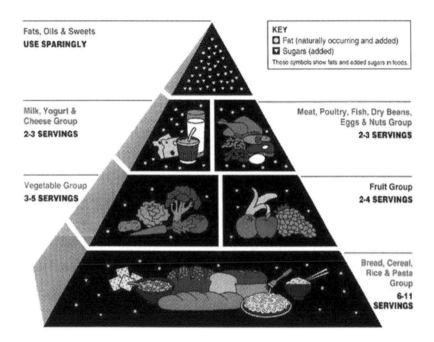

The images above should be shocking to you. If you are an average American and eating these calories as your primary "food," then you should realize that you are following suit with 100 years of conditioning. My recommendation is to reject your conditioning and related eating behavior and take ownership of your brain's corrupted pleasure/happiness system.

Many people feel guilty about their dietary desires and cravings, sometimes not so accurately called an addiction. No one should feel guilty about wanting these foods – this is because, unless you are the extremely rare person, we all desire one or more of these foods.

Action plan to combat food propaganda
Here is the simplest action plan you can engage in regarding the information in this chapter. *Anger* is a good emotion to muster upon discovering that you have been conditioned to eat pro-inflammatory foods, become obese, and then dependent on a slew of medications. This healthy anger can be used as ammunition to

help reject any cravings you may have for these foods and set yourself free, and also protect those you love from eating these foods.

You can also watch and share two YouTube videos I created on the topic of food propaganda.

Food Propaganda from 1912-1950
Food Propaganda - after 1950, present, and future

Action plan for dealing with food urges, food-related suffering, and happiness
Many of the remaining chapters in this book will delve into this topic in more detail. At this point, the best mindset to develop is to recognize that life is difficult and filled with suffering to varying degrees at different times. Understand that happiness is a transient state and that "not being unhappy" is a far more achievable goal to pursue. Regarding food, its purpose is to *nourish* and sustain you; NOT to make you happy.

The "food is pleasure" mindset allows brain physiology, emotions, genes, and primordial factors to take over and when this happens, it is virtually impossible to prevent oneself from becoming fat and obese, and eventually sick and diseased, which is a state of perpetual unhappiness. This mindset must be guarded against and eliminated. It is easier to avoid inflammatory foods that promote weight gain when it is understood that the suffering from eating them far outweighs the normal level of stress, strain, and suffering most people deal with on a daily basis.

When I was growing up, my parents stopped us from regularly experiencing the "happiness" of dessert eating, as it was a rare occurrence to have dessert – the same was true for most of the other kids I grew up with. When I left for college, I was amazed to see what people ate and how easily people gained 10-20 pounds their first year in college, which continued thereafter. Their parents were not there to put the brakes on the drive to overeat dietary crack.

Each of us must cultivate a state of dietary crack mindfulness to suppress or eliminate the consumption of such calories. Engaging in activities you love is also important because it reduces the need for food pleasure. Try to orient your life so you can engage in these activities on a daily basis.

References
1. https://theconversation.com/the-manipulation-of-the-american-mind-edward-bernays-and-the-birth-of-public-relations-44393
2. https://www.smithsonianmag.com/history/how-woodrow-wilsons-propaganda-machine-changed-american-journalism-180963082/
3. Curtis, A. The Century of the Self. https://topdocumentaryfilms.com/the-century-of-the-self/

Chapter 3
Our obesogenic Environment

The cover of this book states that you can learn to control the eating beast within. This starts with understanding the obesogenic environment. Obesogenic means obesity-promoting, and we absolutely live in a weight-gain environment. Our modern living environment ceaselessly tempts us to overeat and avoid physical activity.[1]

Body weight categories
Normal weight, overweight, and obesity categories are based on body mass index (BMI). You can determine your BMI at this NIH page:

https://www.nhlbi.nih.gov/health/educational/lose_wt/BMI/bmica lc.htm?source=quickfitnesssolutions

Here are the BMI categories:
Underweight = < 18.5
Normal weight = 18.5 - 24.9
Overweight = 25 - 29.9
Obesity = 30 or greater

Well-muscled people argue that BMI is inaccurate, as they often have a BMI of 28 or more. The way to determine if your BMI is an accurate marker of excess body fat is to correlate it with waist/hip ratio. This was described in Chapter 9 of *The DeFlame Diet* book. For women, the waist/hip ratio should be less than .8, and for men, less than .95.

For most people, if they are overweight or obese, they will have an elevated BMI and waist/hip ratio. Well-muscled people should focus on waist/hip ratio and not BMI.

In the recent past

When I was a child in the 1960's, some people were overweight, but it was the very rare person who was obese. The environment then was far less obesogenic compared to today. People walked from place to place, walked up stairs, and worked in their yards as part of their normal lifestyle, each of which can be easily avoided today.

Not all, but most people engaged in additional recreational activities, such as running, hiking, swimming, calisthenics, and other sporting activities. Jack LaLanne was the fitness inspiration in America and viewers of his television show were encouraged to exercise along with Jack, and both my mother and grandmother did. There were few gyms for people to go to, save for the rare body building gym, and yet children and adults mostly maintained normal body weight due to engaging in the previously mentioned activities. When we came home from school, most of the kids would run around and play outside until dinner, and sometimes even after dinner. Today is very different, wherein many kids are in front of some form of technology while snacking, when they should be outside running around and being active.

People knew to curb their snacking and dessert eating. When I was growing up, we used to ask what was for dessert...the answer was, "nothing, eat more dinner." Going out to dinner was a luxury that few people I knew engaged in, which also reduced the likelihood of eating dessert.

Today's obesogenic environment

Today, people regularly pig out at restaurants and the servers push appetizers and desserts, both of which drive caloric needs beyond that which is already exceeded by high-calorie meals.

Calorie "pushers" are everywhere. In airports, when I get a bottle of water I am always asked whether I forgot to also buy candy or snacks...like I really *forgot* to buy a candy bar. In the airplane, flight attendants walk by and throw cookies and pretzels at all the passengers in the main cabin. If you are in first class, you get a greater option of calories along with endless beer and wine if you choose.

Stop for gas on the highway and all you see inside the station is a sea of calories made from sugar, flour, and refined oils, along with seemingly endless options of sugar-laden beverages. At all grocery stores, there are aisles of "foods" that are made from sugar, flour, and refined oil.

The above briefly describes the obesogenic environment in which we all live. If we do not live in a "mindful" state, it is nearly impossible to avoid being overweight or obese.

References
1. Berthoud HR. The neurobiology of food intake in an obesogenic environment. Proc Nutr Soc. 2012;71(4):478-87.

Chapter 4
Mindfulness as "the" weapon against weight gain

Mindfulness is a very useful word to understand when it comes to life in general, but especially when dealing with temptation of all kinds, and in the case of this book, the obvious temptation we are dealing with is overeating. Here are two definitions of mindfulness:

> 1. the quality or state of being conscious or aware of something.

> 2. a mental state achieved by focusing one's awareness on the present moment, while calmly acknowledging and accepting one's feelings, thoughts, and bodily sensations, used as a therapeutic technique.

Most people eat in a fashion that is absolutely mindLESS rather than mindful. I notice this no matter where there is food in a public place (mall, movie theatre, restaurant, etc.), but it is especially obvious to me at airports and on airplanes. We are basically caged, so to speak, in the terminal or plane, and the easiest way to distract oneself and feel some pleasure is to eat stuff that tastes good. I feel this pull strongly in my own body, which I mostly resist. This experience has taught me that the drive to eat is very strong in me, and I spend my professional life in this domain, meaning that knowledge about nutrition does not impact the emotional/primordial drive to eat. A state of mindfulness is required. So, for those who spend little time thinking about nutrition, inflammation, and the behavioral and primordial forces that govern eating as I do, they are essentially hopelessly helpless in the battle to maintain proper bodyweight unless they develop dietary mindfulness and further make "not being unhappy" a goal.

Several years ago, I noticed that people became more mindful when they ate with me at a convention table. They thought I was going to judge them, but that was not the case at all. I know how difficult it is to stop the eating beast within and how powerless most people are, so I am not judgmental. What happened to these people at the table was that they became more mindful about their own eating because they were thinking that I was going to judge them. In other words, I functioned as the catalyst for their mindfulness in that moment. The key is to generate dietary mindfulness on your own and make it a way of life.

When I was a senior in college, I weighed about 170 pounds, which is what I weigh today. In order to maintain my college weight almost 40 years later, I have to be mindful of my calorie intake. I weighed almost 190 at one point and this was because I was working long hours sitting and was not mindful of my caloric intake.

In some form or another, most of us have been told that in order to succeed at anything, "you must care" (be mindful) about whatever it is that you wish to achieve. I have experienced this fact of life in many ways. If I cared in school, I did well. At times, I had to talk myself into liking and caring about a class in order to do well. If I did NOT care, I would be happy with a C or D. If I did care, a C or D would be very disturbing. One of my favorite classes in undergraduate college was an exercise physiology class. I got a B+ and was bothered because I loved the class and cared about getting an A.

Marriage - If you want to have a successful marriage, you must care and be mindful. You have to think about the other person a great deal and properly consider their needs in order for the relationship to last in a meaningful fashion.

Sports - If you want to be good at any sporting activity, you must care about it. I made it a goal to become a scratch golfer at one point. A "scratch golfer" refers to someone who scores, on average, par or below par. I cared deeply about this goal. I managed to shoot 73 several times and missed shooting par for legitimate reasons and not because I choked. But then I realized that my motor skills were not good enough to become a scratch golfer without devoting a huge amount of practice hours. I also came to grips with the fact that I did not have the needed hours to devote to this goal, so I gave it up. In other words, I stopped caring about it. Now I play golf whenever I have the chance and do not levy judgment against myself when I play poorly.

Weight management - When it comes to weight loss and maintaining the weight loss, you absolutely *must care* and be mindful. Important to understand is that it takes effort to care and to maintain the weight loss mindset throughout one's life. If you stop being mindful, body weight will accumulate.

What causes us to "not care" and be less mindful?
Stressful events that are distracting lead to a lack of mindfulness and the next thing we know, we are eating foods that we know we should not and in amounts that are far too great. So, when stress enters our lives, we have to ramp up the mindfulness during the period of heightened stress to be able to maintain proper weight and related good behaviors.

Chapter 5
Goals

Goal setting helps to put constraints upon our brain so we can behave in accordance with our goals. Goals help make us mindful and less attached emotional swings that we will inevitably go through in life.

Please take out a sheet of paper and write down your goals. Try to make this as personal as possible for you. Here are some examples:

Body weight goal:

Waist circumference goal:

Clothes size fitting goal:

Longevity goal:

Disease reduction goals:

Health promotion goals:

Activity goals:

I listed multiple anti-inflammation goals in *The DeFlame Diet* book. See Tables 1-4 in Chapter 9, which can be tracked throughout a lifetime to help keep the flame under control.

When humans seriously put their minds on a goal, our lives can change. Achieving serious goals requires mental and behavioral changes that we would not normally experience without the goal or ideal in mind. It is important to understand that the goal itself is not relevant or life changing. Mentally committing to the goal(s) appears be the key ingredient.

Recall the story of my brother Tom in the introduction of this book. He lost 150 pounds in less than a year because he was deeply committed to this goal. He was also committed to no longer needing blood pressure medication, and a reduction in pain and better management of other symptoms of his dystonia, all of which he achieved. His steadfast dedication to his goals is what made him successful in reaching them. Continued dedication to his goals is why he is able to maintain them, so he doesn't suffer more than he has to with his chronic health condition.

When it comes to losing weight, most people can initially do it because they commit to the goal. Regaining the lost weight is very common, and it is not because diets don't work. It is because people give up on their weight loss/management commitment, which allows the influence of all the weight-gain promoters discussed in this book to be released with a vengeance. The outcome is that people will often regain their lost weight and more.

A pain-free life
A pain-free life is a great goal because when we are pain-free, we are released from a source of misery that can be incapacitating.

There are multiple reasons why pain develops. Too much stress, a lack of sleep, sedentary living, and a pro-inflammatory diet all predispose one to develop chronic pain after injury. These are the same factors that promote obesity.

In recent years, research has revealed that obesity promotes most chronic diseases, including musculoskeletal pain. Overweight and obese individuals are more likely to have back pain, disc herniation, joint pain, tendon pain, widespread pain (commonly called fibromyalgia), and headaches.[1] Obesity is also associated with depression and depressed people tend to have chronic aches and pains.

I have met countless people who explained to me that their aches and pains completely disappeared after they went on an anti-inflammatory diet and lost the extra body fat. This does not happen to everyone, but essentially everyone does experience less pain to varying degrees. Everyone feels physically and mentally better after losing weight and for some people, depression completely goes away.

1. Seaman DR. Body mass index and musculoskeletal pain: is there a connection? Chiropractic Man Ther. 2013;21:15.

Chapter 6
The calorie issue

The "calorie" has become a confusing issue for some reason. I cannot exactly put my finger on the precise nature of confusion, but it seems that people think that eating any sugar at all will make them gain weight. This is simply not true, when considered from the "total" daily calorie perspective.

The following information freaks out some people, while it can set others free. Consider the fact that you can lose weight by eating only desserts and reverse diabetes by eating double cheeseburgers as the primary calorie source. Below is a DeFlame Nutrition YouTube video I created on this topic:

DeFlame with Twinkies and Double Cheeseburgers AND lose weight and even reverse diabetes?

Please understand that I am not suggesting that one should eat desserts and double cheeseburgers; the point is that total calories are the most important factor for achieving and maintaining body weight. There is a popular notion that one absolutely does not need to count calories to lose weight – this is true for some but not for others. It is only true if you eat mostly vegetation, which is low in calories. If you eat no sugar or flour, a moderate amount of vegetation, and lots of nuts, cheese, avocados, and heavy cream poured over fruit, there is a good chance you will have a high calorie diet and promote weight gain.

Almost everybody who is trying to lose weight will have moments of cheating. So long as these moments do not lead to exceeding caloric needs, weight loss can continue and be maintained. Do not get down on yourself if you find yourself putting ice cream and cake in your mouth on occasion.

Calories and metabolic rate

It is a fact that if you eat less calories and lose body fat, your body metabolism, or metabolic rate, will slow down. This is often looked upon as a bad thing, but it is an excellent thing. This means that you can eat less calories and easily maintain body weight once you reach your desired goal. The slowing of body metabolism is a normal healthy response that allows us to maintain body weight with less calories.

IMPORTANT – if you lose your state of eating mindfulness, then it is true that you can accumulate body fat faster if metabolism has been slowed due to caloric restriction. This only means that you must sustain a state of food/eating mindfulness.

Calories and body fat reduction

The foods we eat contain protein, fat, and carbohydrate, which we can convert to a substance called adenosine triphosphate (ATP), which is the body's energy source. There are three pathways involved in energy production, which are called glycolysis, the Kreb's Cycle, and the electron transport chain. The latter two generate the most energy, so we want them working optimally. Overeating carbohydrate, especially sugar and flour, shifts energy production away from Kreb's and electron transport, toward glycolysis, which means less fat utilization for energy production and so, less body fat reduction.[1] Clearly, we do not want this. In contrast, eating less carbohydrate and more fat supports optimal activity of Kreb's and electron transport, which we definitely want because that is where fat utilization for energy occurs, which optimizes body fat reduction.

A study of overweight men and women compared two diets that contained 1500 calories.[2] The high carbohydrate diet contained 56% percent of calories from carbohydrate, 24% from fat, and 20% from protein. The permitted foods included whole grains (breads, cereals, and pastas), fruit/fruit juices, vegetables, vegetable oils, low-fat dairy and lean meat products. Notice that while this diet contained carbohydrate from grains and fruit, no sugar or white flour were permitted.

The low carbohydrate diet contained 12% percent of calories from carbohydrate, 59% from fat, and 28% from protein. They permitted beef, poultry, fish, eggs, oils, and heavy cream; moderate amounts of hard cheeses, low carbohydrate vegetables, and salad dressings; and small amounts of nuts, nut butters and seeds.

Not surprisingly, each group lost weight as they were both low in calories. Body fat loss was slightly better with the low carbohydrate diet because, as stated above, eating less carbohydrate and more fat improves body fat loss. Both diets were anti-inflammatory; however, the low carbohydrate/high fat diet was more anti-inflammatory. The low carbohydrate diet in this study was ketogenic and contained less than 50 grams of carbohydrate per day. My impression is that for those who do not wish to eat a ketogenic diet, it is best to limit carbohydrate consumption to no more than 100 grams per day. However, the guiding dietary principle should be achieving normal markers of inflammation.

As I stated in Chapter 1 of this book, my view is to choose foods that suit your mind and body, and allow you to achieve and maintain normal makers of inflammation as outlined in Chapter 9 of *The DeFlame Diet* book.

Should you fast?

Fasting has become much more popular in recent years, which I find interesting for the following reason. Many people have a hard time avoiding unhealthy pro-inflammatory calories and eating more anti-inflammatory calories. Fasting is eating no calories at all, which leads me to think that the average person should first learn to do a "dietary crack" fast before moving to actual fasting. The reason for looking at it like this should be obvious. If people do not learn to avoid dietary crack first, then after a fast, they will likely resort to eating dietary crack again. The outcome is the yoyo cycling of weight loss and weight gain that is all too common.

Perhaps the best way to combine a dietary crack fast and regular fasting is to engage in what is called time-restricted feeding (TRF).[3] There is both a mental and physiologic benefit from TRF, in which one can only eat during a designated 8-hour time period. For example, when I am doing TRF, I eat only between 12 noon and 8 PM. Then I do not eat from 8 PM until 12 noon the next day. Water is allowed and black coffee in the morning, or regular or green tea if that is preferred. As one adapts to the 16:8 cycle, then it is easier to extend the fasting time, while only eating anti-inflammatory foods during the feeding period until you do a total fast if you wish to move in that direction.

The mental benefit of a 16:8 TRF lifestyle is that you absolutely have to be mindful to not eat during those hours, a time-period wherein the average non-TRF person can consume 1000 calories or more. So, you have to control any urges and force yourself to wait out the 16-hour "fasting" period, which you can make longer if you wish. Let's say you eat no calories until 2 PM; then you have a 6-hour eating window.

The physical benefits of TRF is that you will decrease fat mass, maintain or increase muscle mass, and promote a DeFlamed state. I am a big supporter of TRF; however, if you cannot do it, make sure to keep your caloric intake appropriate and focus on eating anti-inflammatory foods. I think it is best to not stress about absolutely being in ketosis or doing a perfect 16:8 TRF program. The easiest, unemotional way to eat is to make the achievement and maintenance of normal markers of inflammation the goal, as outlined in Chapter 9 of the *The DeFlame Diet* book.

References
1. Sarto R, Jackson MJ, Squillace C et al. Adaptive metabolic response to 4 weeks of sugar-sweetened beverage consumption in healthy, lightly active individuals and chronic high glucose availability in primary human myotubes. Eur J Nutr. 2013;52:937-48.

2. Forsythe CE, Phinney SD, Fernandez ML et al. Comparison of low fat and low carbohydrate diets on circulating fatty acid composition and markers of inflammation. Lipids. 2008;43:65-77.

3. Moro T, Tinsley G, Bianco A, et al. Effects of eight weeks of time-restricted feeding (16/8) on basal metabolism, maximal strength, body composition, inflammation, and cardiovascular risk factors. J Transl Med. 2016;14:290

Chapter 7
Sustained weight management

I commonly hear something similar to this: "I go on a liquid diet, shake diet, paleo diet, DeFlame diet, etc., but when I go off the diet, I gain weight." This is kind of a foolish statement, because of course you will gain weight if you stop minding your caloric intake. For people who think like this, they need to ask themselves the following question: Why am I going off the diet or not transitioning properly?

In short, the average person does not plan for life after weight loss. If you do not understand that we live in an obesogenic environment and combat the eating stimuli that are everywhere, you will gain weight. Without a persevering state of eating mindfulness, you will gain weight. Without short and long-term goals that are body weight dependent, you will gain weight. Without keeping track of calories, you will gain weight.

Sustained weight management requires that you be mentally present in a vigilant fashion. The remaining chapters examine additional factors that you must be aware of to keep your body weight under control.

Chapters 8-17 are about why we are fat and outline the multiple factors that drive the eating beast within us all. You can view the eating beast as an alter ego, similar to Dr. Jekyll and Mr. Hyde. The eating beast is Mr. Hyde-like and needs to be controlled.

Chapter 8
Why we are fat – we eat too fast

In 2010, researchers concluded that, "the warning we were given as children that wolfing down your food will make you fat may in fact have a physiological explanation." The study demonstrated that eating the same meal over 30 minutes instead of 5 minutes lead to an earlier feeling of satiety, which correlated to the release of anti-hunger hormones. In other words, those who ate the meal slowly felt more full and were less hungry.[1] Multiple other studies have led to similar conclusions.[2-6]

The issue appears to be particularly problematic in terms of weight gain, when high calorie, low fiber foods are consumed rapidly.[5] Eating too fast also promotes high blood glucose levels and lowers HDL cholesterol, which are markers of chronic inflammation, and this occurs no matter if one is obese or not.[6]

Eating too fast is extremely common and an obvious promoter of weight gain and chronic inflammation. I witness fast eating on airplanes, in airports, at conventions, at work, and in restaurants. I also catch myself at times eating too quickly. Starting today, force yourself to eat more slowly. It is the first and easiest step toward proper weight management.

References
1. Kokkinos A et al. Eating slowly increases the postprandial response of the anorexogenic gut hormones, peptide YY and glucagon-like peptide-1. J Clin Endocrinol Metab. 2010;95:333-37.
2. Angelopoulos T et al. The effect of slow spaced eating on hunger and satiety in overweight and obese patients with type 2 diabetes. BMJ Open Diabetes Res Care. 2014;2:e000013.
3. Andrade AM et al. Eating slowly led to decreases in energy within meals in healthy women. J Am Diet Assoc. 2008;108:1186-91.
4. Salazar Vazquez BY. Control of overweight and obesity in childhood through education in meal time habits. The 'good manners for a healthy future' programme. Pediatric Obesity. 2016;11:484-90.

5. Karl JP et al. Independent and combined effects of eating rate on energy density and on energy intake, appetite, gut hormones. Obesity. 2013;21:E244-52.

6. Lee KS et al. Eating rate is associated with cardiometabolic risk factors in Korean adults. Nutr Metab Cardiovasc Dis. 2013;23:635-41.

Chapter 9
Why we are fat – the instinctual drive to overeat

Do we really have an instinctual drive to overeat? I do not know if it has been officially established as scientific fact, however, operationally it is certainly true and quite observable. We certainly do have an instinctual drive to eat and to absolutely eat calorie-rich foods. Without eating we would die, so eating is an absolute biological imperative and humans will riot and revolt for food. For example, in part, the French Revolution was driven by food scarcity.

Pre-agricultural humans were hunter-gatherers. They had to literally exercise for food. The same held true when people farmed for food, because farming involves exercise. The pre-agricultural and pre-industrial eras were a very different world compared to today from many perspectives and the availability of food is no exception. Consider the following perspective from Paleolithic nutrition researchers O'Keefe and Cordain[1]:

> "Our cravings for calorie-dense foods, such as fats, sweets, and starches, are legacies of our Paleolithic ancestors, who sought these foods because they conferred positive survival value in an environment in which these food types were scarce. These cravings betray us in our modern world, where calorie-dense foods are abundant and inexpensive, and most people die of caloric excess manifested as obesity, the metabolic syndrome, hypertension, and cardiovascular disease."

So, if you crave calorie-dense foods, consider yourself a normal human. These were prized foods historically because they promoted human survival, which means the powerful urges to eat and eat and eat these foods is completely normal. The problem is that in modern society these foods are no longer scarce, which means we must control our instinctual drive to gorge on these foods and rather, behave as if they were *not* so plentiful. Of course, this is easier said than done, but you must nonetheless develop a mindset that helps to make this behavior a habit.

Your body wants you fat

In nature, animals always weigh more before winter begins for the purpose of dealing with food scarcity during winter. Come springtime, animals are leaner and in need of food, which is now naturally more plentiful. Animals eat and gain weight during the spring through fall in preparation for another winter. Human bodies work on the same natural rhythm. Clearly, a person with added fat can live longer without food compared to a thin person. Thus, an important primal instinct is to gain weight for the purpose of dealing with a coming famine or winter...so, for practical purposes, you should accept that your body wants you fat.

Your desire to eat and eat is not unique to you or family members, just because many of you may be overweight. Eating and overeating are instinctual drives for self-preservation that is consistent among most, if not all, species in the animal kingdom. Bad genes are rarely the cause of excessive weight gain despite this excuse people like to use. It is much more likely that bad eating habits within families is the cause of generational obesity, which is misperceived as a genetic problem.

To remain lean in a food environment wherein there is an abundance of available calories on nearly every street corner means that we must battle against our self-preservation instincts that will always be there for as long as we live. Operationally, this means that every human on earth would be fat if we let our instincts completely dominate our eating behavior. So, without the awareness that being overweight is essentially an instinctual drive associated with self-preservation, people can misinterpret their "overeating problem" as a type of personal mental problem that is somehow unique to them. While this is not at all true, it is a reasonable misinterpretation to have if one does not understand that our bodies want us fat for survival purposes.

Since our bodies want us fat, you must accept the fact that your body wants you fat. And the way to address this human challenge is to psychologically step in with your will power and mindfulness, and dominate the eating process with logic, rather than letting the emotional eating instincts go wild. This means clearing your fridge, freezer, cabinets, and hiding places of all pro-inflammatory foods. Only anti-inflammatory foods should be kept in your home.

My suggestion is to not dramatize the fact that your body wants you fat – it is just normal physiology. Be logical. Sit back and observe in yourself how the instinctual drive pushes you to eat calorie-dense pro-inflammatory foods, and then exert dominion over these drives. Make it a goal to eat anti-inflammatory foods and exercise regularly to achieve and maintain normal levels of the inflammatory markers in Tables 1-4 of Chapter 9 of *The DeFlame Diet* book.

References
1. O'Keefe JH, Cordain L. Cardiovascular disease resulting from a diet and lifestyle at odds with our Paleolithic genome: how to become a 21st-century hunter-gatherer. Mayo Clin Proc. 2004;79:101-108.

Chapter 10
Why we are fat – too much stress

Stress and eating

The chemistry of stress is complex and researchers are still unraveling all the details. Fortunately, we know enough to describe the relationship between stress with eating in a practical fashion that we can apply to our lives.

Dr. Hans Selye, who discovered the stress response, made it clear that stress is the response to stressors, which can affect us differently. A stressor to you may not be a stressor to me; however, when we do experience stress, the chemistry is mostly identical among all individuals. And stress is very common within the United States population, such that the American Psychological Association indicates that most Americans suffer from moderate stress.

You have likely heard the terms "stress eating" and "self-medication with comfort foods" during times of stress. In fact, researchers have identified changes in body metabolism that occur during stress eating.[1-5] When we are stressed, a hormone called ghrelin is released from the stomach and pancreas. It quickly reaches the brain where it stimulates the appetite centers in a region called the hypothalamus.

It would be great if ghrelin stimulated the desire for us to eat anti-inflammatory foods such as vegetables, meat, and fish, but quite to the contrary. Instead, ghrelin stimulates us to eat highly palatable, calorie-dense comfort foods that are rich in sugar, flour, and fat (dietary crack), which would not have been a problem when these foods were not readily available as they are in our modern times.

There is a physiological benefit of ghrelin release that should be understood. Once ghrelin hits the brain, it helps to reduce depression.[1] So important is this effect that ghrelin has been described as a survival hormone.[2] In particular, this would have been advantageous when pre-modern era man was forced to deal with various stressors. The released ghrelin would help prevent depression and despair and allow people to persevere. The anti-depressant effect of ghrelin would have helped people to stay engaged in whatever task/activity they were involved with that likely involved efforts to survive in difficult environments without food stores, restaurants, modern luxuries, and appliances.

The ghrelin-comfort food connection would have had little impact during pre-modern times, as dietary crack calories were not readily available, so there would have been no dietary crack to crave. Our current challenge is to deal with ghrelin release during stress in an obesogenic environment while we are sedentary and physically inactive. This means that when we get stressed and ghrelin pushes us to eat dietary crack, we must pause, be mindful, and realize that we are just in a "ghrelin moment" that will pass. Instead of reaching for dietary crack, we must get mentally engaged in meaningful work, family activities, physical activities, or exercise.

As described in the previous chapter, we instinctually crave calorie-dense foods in the absence of stress to make sure we have enough body fat to get through periods of food scarcity. Then, when we become chronically stressed by the hustle and bustle of modern life, ghrelin stimulates the overt craving of these same foods. This means that to maintain a proper body weight, we have to regularly contend with primordial eating drives coupled with stress-induced eating metabolism. You can see why it is so important to develop caloric mindfulness and adhere to eating rules such as the 16:8 time-restricted feeding approach discussed earlier in Chapter 6.

Stress and fat gain chemistry
As most live with at least moderate stress, the problems associated with chronic stress should not be taken lightly. Not only does

stress, by virtue of ghrelin release, push us to overeat pro-inflammatory foods, the chemistry of stress itself is a chemistry of "weight gain."

Major stress hormones include cortisol, adrenalin, renin, growth hormone and glucagon.[6-8] Cortisol is produced by our adrenal glands. People can also take cortisol as a medication (prednisone, prednisolone, and methylprednisolone) for inflammatory conditions such as rheumatorid arthritis and other autoimmune diseases.

One of the outcomes of excess cortisol produced by the body due to stress or from taking cortisol medications is insulin resistance.[8] This means that muscles will not respond to insulin properly, leading to elevated levels of circulating insulin. Elevated insulin levels promote the conversion of glucose from refined carbohydrates into fat.[9] This is such an important obesity issue that researchers are trying to develop drugs to reduce the body's production of cortisol for the purpose of reducing insulin resistance to treat obesity and diabetes.[10]

How would you know if you are moving toward insulin resistance and increasing your risk of growing your body fat mass? Researchers explain that stress-induced insulin resistance can manifest as[6,7]:

1. high blood glucose
2. increased triglycerides
3. reduced HDL cholesterol
4. elevation of blood pressure
5. abdominal obesity

If you quickly take a look at Table 3 in Chapter 9 of *The DeFlame Diet* book, you will see that these are the markers of the metabolic syndrome. This means that stress-induced insulin resistance and inflammatory diet-induced insulin resistance work together to promote body fatness. It turns out that a lack of sleep does the same thing, which will be described in the next chapter.

Unfortunately, there is an additional fat-promoting effect of cortisol and insulin. Each hormone stimulates the brain to promote the consumption of tasty pro-inflammatory foods.[11,12] What makes this situation worse is that the pleasurable experience of tasting pro-inflammatory foods temporarily reduces activity in the stress-response system, so one feels happy during the eating event and less stressed out, which serves to reinforce the habit of overeating inflammatory foods.[13]

Avoiding stressors

Life is stressful, so to suggest that the average person can become stress-free is not realistic. Some stressors are unavoidable, such as those related to work, finances, holidays, and family issues. Other stressors are absolutely avoidable and they are unique from one person to the next and should be categorized as, "choices that unnecessarily complicate our lives." Take stock of yourself and your life to identify these choices/stressors and then do your best to avoid them completely.

Exercise as an antidote to stress

When we feel stressed, this mostly translates into depression and/or anxiety and most people reach for pro-inflammatory dietary crack. Instead of reaching for dietary crack, we instead need to choose exercise, which has many beneficial effects:

- Generates an immediate reward/pleasure response[14]
- Promotes a general feeling of well-being[15]
- Appetite suppressive effects[16,17]
- Anti-depressive effects[15,18-20]
- Anti-anxiety effects[15,21,22]
- Anti-stress effects[23]
- Anti-inflammatory effects[24]

Identifying the specific level of exercise intensity and duration is the trick to achieving these desired effects of exercise. For me, it is a fairly intense level of exercise for 30-60 minutes, which includes intermittent rest periods.

I identified my intensity level by accident a few years ago on a Saturday morning when I needed to leave the house by 10:30 AM to catch a plane. I got up before 6 AM with the intention of exercising around 7 AM, but I got lost in what I was working on and ended up exercising from 9 to 10 AM. Then I jumped in the shower and was out the door by 10:30. While driving to the airport, I realized that I was hungry before exercising, but was not anymore, and this continued until after 12 noon. So, I started to work with this and quickly identified that whatever time of day I exercised at the intensity needed for appetite suppression, that is when I also get the exercise reward/pleasure response and an improved feeling of well-being.

Another important benefit of exercise is that it helps to reset the body weight set point to a lower weight, which enables one to more easily maintain lower body weights. This topic will be discussed more in Chapter 12.

References
1. Chuang JC, PerelloM, Sakata I, et al. Ghrelin mediates stress-induced food-reward behavior in mice. J Clin Invest 2011;121(7):2684–92.
2. Mani BK, Zigman JM. Ghrelin as a survival hormone. Trends Endocrinol Metab. 2017;28:843-54.
3. Dallman MF, Pecoraro NC, la Fleur SE. Chronic stress and comfort foods: self-medication and abdominal obesity. Brain Behav Immun 2005;19:275–80.
4. Adam TC, Epe ES. Stress, eating and the reward system. Physiol Behav 2007;91:449–58.
5. Maniam J, Morris MJ. The link between stress and feeding behaviour. Neuropharmacol 2012;63:97–110.
6. Black PH. The inflammatory response is an integral part of the stress response: implications for atherosclerosis, insulin resistance, type II diabetes and metabolic syndrome X. Brain Behav Immun 2003;17:350–64.
7. Black PH. The inflammatory consequences of psychologic stress: relationship to insulin resistance, obesity, atherosclerosis and diabetes mellitus, type II. Med Hypoth. 2006;67:879-91.

8. Tchernof A, Després JP. Pathophysiology of human visceral obesity: an update. Physiol Rev. 2013;93(1):359-404.

9. Kersten S. Mechanisms of nutritional and hormonal regulation of lipogenesis. EMBO Rep. 2001;21(41):282-86.

10. Joharapurkar A, Dhanesha N, Shah G, Kharul R, Jain M. 11β-Hydroxysteroid dehydrogenase type 1: potential therapeutic target for metabolic syndrome. Pharmacol Rep. 2012;64(5):1055-65.

11. Dallman MF, Pecoraro N, Akana SF, et al. Chronic stress and obesity: a new view of "comfort food". Proc Natl Acad Sci U S A. 2003;100(20):11696-701.

12. Dallman MF, Warne JP, Foster MT, Pecoraro NC. Glucocorticoids and insulin both modulate caloric intake through actions on the brain. J Physiol. 2007 Sep 1;583(Pt 2):431-6.

13. Dallman MF. Stress-induced obesity and the emotional nervous system. Trends Endocrinol Metab. 2010;21(3):159-65.

14. Salmon P. Effects of physical exercise on anxiety, depression, and sensitivity to stress: a unifying theory. Clin Psychol Rev. 2001;21:33061

15. Scully D, Kremer J, Meade MM, Graham R, Dudgeon K. Physical exercise and psychological well being: a critical review. Brit J Sports Med. 1998;32:111-120.

16. Martins C, Robertson MD, Morgan LM. Effects of exercise and restrained eating behavior on appetite control. Proc Nutr Soc. 2008;67:28–41

17. Martins C, Kulseng B, King NA, Holst JJ, Blundell JE. The effects of exercise-induced weight loss on appetite-related peptides and motivation to eat. J Clin Endocrinol Metab. 2010;95(4):1609–1616

18. Babyak M, Blumenthal JA, Herman S, et al. Exercise treatment for major depression: maintenance of therapeutic benefit at 10 months. Psychosom Med. 2000;62(5):633-8.

19. Blumenthal JA, Babyak MA, Doraiswamy PM, et al. Exercise and pharmacotherapy in the treatment of major depressive disorder. Psychosom Med. 2007;69(7):587-96.

20. Blumenthal JA, Smith PJ, Hoffman BM. Is Exercise a Viable Treatment for Depression? ACSMs Health Fit J. 2012;16(4):14-21.

21. Petruzzello SJ et al. A meta-analysis on the anxiety-reducing effects of acute and chronic exercise. Sports Med. 1991;11:143-82.

22. Schoenfeld TJ et al. Physical exercise prevents stress-induced activation of granule neurons and enhances local inhibitory mechanisms in the dentate gyrus. J Neurosci. 2013;33:7770-77.

23. Puterman E et al. Physical activity moderates stressor-induced rumination on cortisol reactivity. Psychosom Med. 2011;73:604-11.

24. Flynn MG, McFarlin BK, Markofski MM. The anti-inflammatory actions of exercise training. Am J Lifestyle Med. 2007;1:220-35.

Chapter 11
Why we are fat – a lack of sleep

If you have trouble getting a good night's sleep, you are not alone. According to the Centers for Disease Control and Prevention, inadequate sleep is a public health epidemic.[1] Historically, a lack of sleep was merely viewed as a source of daytime fatigue. A great deal more is now known about the devastating impact that reduced sleep has on body function. Reduced sleep:

- Promotes inflammation[2-4]
- Promotes aches and pains[5]
- Promotes insulin resistance[6-9]
- Increases hunger and food intake[10]
- Prevents weight loss efforts[11]
- Promotes depression[12,13]

The precise amount of sleep we need to prevent these untoward effects depends on the individual; however, researchers have identified that 6-9 hours of sleep is the appropriate range for most people. Less than 6 hours or more than 9 hours of sleep increases risk of pain expression. Less than 6 hours of sleep prevents weight loss and metabolic risk factor reduction, and promotes obesity.[8,11]

Of importance to note, we do not need 6 hours of straight sleep per night. We need at least 6 hours during a 24-hour cycle. Research has indeed identified that napping allows us to catch up.[14] Napping has also been studied in first-year medical school residents who are notoriously sleep deprived. Napping improved cognitive function and reduced attention related errors.[15]

As noted above, reduced sleep is a promoter of depression.[12,13] This is problematic because depression is a risk factor for obesity.[16] This means that most all of us need to do what we can to make sure we get at least 6 hours of sleep in a 24-hour period.

Important to realize is that if you are not getting adequate sleep, odds favor that your mind will be less attracted to exercise and anti-inflammatory foods, and more attracted to sedentary living and the consumption of dietary crack. You must resist these attractions. Force yourself to engage in physical activity, even if it is just 10 minutes of vigorous exercise, and force yourself to eat anti-inflammatory foods at a calorically appropriate level for you.

Basic things we can do to promote better sleep

A dark room is a key issue for many people. Room temperature is also very important. We appear to sleep best at a room temperature between 60-67 degrees Fahrenheit. If that is too cold, try to get to at least 70 degrees or less. Work with it until you find the coolest temperature that works best for you. My brother Tom provides excellent sleep recommendations in his book, *Diagnosis Dystonia: Navigating the Journey*:

> Make your bedroom reflective of the value you place on sleep. Check your room for noise, light, temperature, or other distractions, including a partner's sleep disruptions such as snoring. Consider using shades that darken the room, a sleep mask to cover your eyes, earplugs, recordings of soothing sounds, and a fan or other device that creates white noise.
>
> Other tips include sticking to a sleep schedule, increasing light exposure during the day, creating a bedtime ritual, reserving your bed for sleeping and sex only, and limiting how much you drink before bed to prevent trips to the bathroom.

Sleep can also be improved by regular exercise.[17,18] A mechanism by which this occurs is via inflammation reduction, which is an especially important goal as we age. As stated earlier in Chapter 1, inflammation levels increase as we age. For many people, this inflammaging process is associated with poor sleep quality that never seems to improve. It turns out that regular moderate exercise improves sleep in 71-year-old subjects.[18] This means that we should exercise throughout life no matter how old we get.

Many people have told me that their sleep has improved significantly by following *The DeFlame Diet*. This improvement has been noticed within the first week for many and within the first month for the majority, unless they have sleep apnea. I published a case history about a patient who suffered with sleep apnea and wore a CPAP device for 10 years.[19] In just 3 months of DeFlaming his diet, he no longer needed the CPAP device, and this success has been maintained since 2004 when the patient was 55 years old.

In short, obesity is significantly correlated to disordered sleep and sleep apnea. As 20% of adults have mild sleep apnea[19], it is very important to achieve and maintain normal body weight.

References
1. CDC . Insufficient sleep is a public health epidemic. Centers for Disease Control. http://www.cdc.gov/Features/dsSleep/
2. Motivala SJ. Sleep and inflammation. psychoneuroimmunology in the context of cardiovascular disease. Ann Behav Med. 2011;42:141–152
3. Mullington JM, Simpson NS, Meier-Ewert HK, Haak M. Sleep loss and inflammation. Best Prac Res Clin Endocrinol Metab. 2010;24:775–784
4. Meier-Ewert HK, Ridker PM, Rifai N, et al. Effect of sleep loss on C-reactive protein, an inflammatory marker of cardiovascular risk. J Am Coll Cardiol. 2004;43:678–683
5. Edwards R, Almeida DM, Klick B, Haythornthwaite JA, Smith MT. Duration of
    sleep contributes to next-day pain report in the general population. Pain. 2008;137:202–207.
6. Lucassen EA, Rother KI, Cizza G. Interacting epidemics? Sleep curtailment, insulin resistance, and obesity. Ann NY Acad Sci. 2012;1264:110–134
7. Morselli L, Leproult R, Balbo M, Spiegel K. Role of sleep duration in the regulation of glucose metabolism and appetite. Best Prac Res Clin Endocrinol Metab. 2010;24:687–702
8. Leproult R, Van Cauter E. Role of sleep and sleep loss in hormonal release and metabolism. Endocr Dev. 2010;17:11–21
9. Knutson KL, Spiegel K, Penev P, van Cauter E. The metabolic consequences of sleep deprivation. Sleep Med Rev. 2007;11:163–178
10. Spiegel K, Tasali E, Penev P, Van Cauter E. Sleep curtailment in healthy young men is associated with decreased leptin levels, elevated ghrelin levels

and increased hunger and appetite. Ann Intern Med. 2004;141:846–850

11. Nedeltcheva AV, Kilkus JM, Imperial J, Schoeller DA, Penev PD. Insufficient sleep undermines dietary efforts to reduce obesity. Ann Int Med. 2010;153:435–441

12. Gangwisch JE, Babiss LA, Malaspina D, Turner JB, Zammit GK, Posner K. Earlier parental set bedtimes as a protective factor against depression and suicidal ideation. Sleep. 2010;33:97–106

13. Chang JJ, Salas J, Habicht K, Pien GW, Stamatikis KA, Brownson RC. The association of sleep duration and depressive symptoms in rural communities of Missouri, Tennessee, and Arkansas. J Rural Health. 2012;28:268–276

14. Pejovic S, Basta M, Vgontzas AN, et al. Effects of recovery sleep after one work week of mild sleep restriction on interleukin-6 and cortisol secretion and daytime sleepiness and performance. Am J Physiol Endocrinol Metab. 2013;305(7):E890-6.

15. Amin MM, Graber M, Ahmad K et al. The effects of a mid-day nap on the neurocognitive performance of first-year medical residents: a controlled interventional pilot study. Acad Med. 2012;87(10):1428-33.

16. Luppino FS, de Wit LM, Bouvy PF, et al. Overweight, obesity, and depression: a systematic review and meta-analysis of longitudinal studies. Arch Gen Psychiatry. 2010;67(3):220–229

17. Santos RV et al. Exercise, sleep, and cytokines: is there a relation? Sleep Med Rev. 2007;11:231-39.

18. Santos RV et al. Moderate exercise training modulates cytokine profile and sleep in elderly people. Cytokine. 2012;60:731-35.

19. Gala TR, Seaman DR. Lifestyle modifications and the resolution of obstructive sleep apnea syndrome: a case report. J Chiro Med. 2011;10:118-25.

Chapter 12

Why we are fat – The paradox of feeling very hungry even though the stomach feels full

After you eat and your stomach feels full, are you still hungry? I am not referring to the ability and desire to keep stuffing oneself. I can always stuff more food in, even when I am full and *not* hungry.

Here is the context of this question. Most people can recall going to a restaurant and having a drink, a salad, bread, and/or perhaps an appetizer before the main course arrives. Most people can also remember during one or all of these times when they, in fact, felt full and no longer hungry before the main course arrived. With this in mind, consider again the following question:

After you eat and your stomach feels full, are you still hungry?

If your stomach is full and you still feel hungry, it is mostly likely because your brain is inflamed and playing tricks on you. In Chapter 13 of *The DeFlame Diet* book, I describe how extra body fat causes inflammation. Circulating levels of inflammatory mediators, such as of high-sensitivity C-reactive protein (hsCRP) and other inflammatory mediators are correlated with weight, BMI, waist circumference, hip circumference, and waist-hip ratio.[1] In other words, the more overweight we become, the more inflamed we become, and this body-wide inflammation directly influences brain function at some point, which leads to the sensation of the stomach feeling very full and still having the sensation of insatiable hunger.

The hypothalamus is the region of the brain that controls hunger. My suggestion is to google the word hypothalamus and click on images. This way you will get many, many images of the hypothalamus. It is a small area in the middle of the brain and it is involved in all the automatic activities in our body, such as hunger, digestion, breathing, heart rate, body temperature, hormonal activity, sleep, and emotional regulation.

When the body becomes progressively inflamed, the hypothalamus loses its ability to respond to two hormones that reduce the sensation of hunger, those being insulin and leptin. Insulin is released by the pancreas, while leptin is released by fat cells. The inflamed hypothalamus is described as being insulin and leptin resistant, because it no longer responds to their anti-hunger messages[2-4], so people feel hungry and keep eating even though they feel full.

Feeling hungry when the stomach is full should be viewed as a metabolic illusion that messes with the human psyche and is a symptom of chronic inflammation. We humans take hunger very seriously – we don't like to feel hungry for very long, and for a good reason. Everyone knows that if you stop eating, you will die. This means that hunger is a powerful primordial drive associated with self-preservation, which means we instinctually act on hunger by eating to survive.

When the body and hypothalamus are inflamed, the feelings of hunger no longer represent the need for calories for self-preservation; in fact, the opposite is true. The illusory "feeling" of hunger, created by an inflamed hypothalamus, is detrimental to our self-preservation because it induces us to overeat and become progressively more inflamed and therefore, we place ourselves at a greater risk of dying younger from a heart attack, cancer, or other chronic disease.

The illusion of feeling hungry even when the stomach feels full will go away. It just takes a little time, which varies from person to person. The first step is to eat only anti-inflammatory foods and consume enough low calorie vegetation to feel full. Initially, one needs to muster all the mental power to respect the feeling of fullness in the stomach and stop eating even though there may still be the "feeling" of hunger. The second step is to exercise at whatever capacity you can tolerate based on one's medical situation. The third step is to track the inflammation markers described in Chapter 9 in *The DeFlame Diet* book. As the markers normalize, inflammation will recede and body physiology can normalize, which means the hypothalamus will register "no longer hungry" after eating. For many people, just the act of eating anti-inflammatory foods to the point of feeling full helps to reduce hunger.

You might be wondering: "How can I figure out if my hypothalamus is inflamed? Is there a test?" This is a very reasonable question; however, at this time there is no diagnostic test that specifically identifies an inflamed hypothalamus. Instead we can operationally determine if the hypothalamus is inflamed or not. Answer this important question again: After a full meal and your stomach "feels" full, are you still hungry?

- If the answer is yes, then your hypothalamus is likely to be inflamed.
- If you answered no, then your hypothalamus is probably not inflamed.

If you have the *The DeFlame Diet* book, go to Chapter 9 and look at the markers in Table 3 and 4. Get the markers measured as soon as you can and keep track of them. The more abnormal inflammation markers you have, the greater the odds are that you have systemic and hypothalamic inflammation, or are moving in that direction. Be very objective about the results and where you stand and then begin to diligently work on the DeFlaming process. Understand that 1/3 of the adult population is of normal weight, which means you can achieve and maintain normal weight if you work at it.

Mindless eating

What if you feel full after eating a meal and you are no longer hungry, and you still keep eating? This is called mindless eating, or pigging out for no reason other than for pleasure or due to stress. Most people are guilty of doing this even if they are lean. I do it as well. So, after a meal, you will need to sit quietly and examine how you feel. Craving dessert does not mean that your hypothalamus is inflamed; remember, craving sweets means that you are a dietary crackhead, like me and most other people.

It is important to understand that pigging out on occasion is no problem, but making it a lifestyle pattern leads to weight gain, chronic inflammation, and hypothalamic inflammation, which then leads to the feeling of hunger even when the stomach feels full. You do not want to get to that state...and if you are already there, it will take 2-4 weeks for it to become a manageable drive that requires ongoing dietary mindfulness. In other words, the "feeling hungry despite being full" experience will typically improve markedly within a month as inflammation subsides and the hypothalamus becomes properly responsive to insulin and leptin; thereafter, people need to be mindful about eating in general and be respectful about the feeling of fullness.

References
1. Park HS, Park LY, Yu R. Relationship of obesity and visceral adiposity with serum concentrations of CRP, TNF-alpha and IL-6. Diabetes Res Clin Pract. 2005;69:29–35.
2. Thaler JP, Schwartz MW. Minireview: inflammation and obesity pathogenesis: the hypothalamus heats up. Endocrinol. 2010;151:4109–15.
3. Thaler JP, Yi CX, Schur EA, et al. Obesity is associated with hypothalamic injury in rodents and humans. J Clin Invest. 2012;122:153–62.
4. Wisse BE, Schwartz MW. Does hypothalamic inflammation cause obesity? Cell Metab. 2009;10:241–2.

Chapter 13
Why we are fat – the battle against
the body weight set point

In the last chapter I described how the body feels hungry even though the stomach feels full. Recall that this occurs because the hypothalamus is no longer able to register the feeling of fullness because it cannot respond to insulin and leptin.

> Researchers explain that these metabolic changes that occur in the hypothalamus due to diet-induced hypothalamic inflammation actually functions to *"increase the defended level of body weight."*[1]

This is one of the most important sentences in this book regarding weight loss. Why would your brain want to "defend" your body weight if you are 40 or more pounds overweight and unhealthy *and* further try to make you get heavier? Believe it or not, the defense of body weight is actually a genius move by the body.

For most of human time on earth, food was not plentiful as it is today. So our innate ability to easily pack on extra body fat that could function as a source of calories in times of food scarcity would increase one's chance of survival.[2] But that was a different era and now food is available on nearly every street corner. Unfortunately, the hypothalamus is unaware of this change in food availability and is still operating as if food is scarce and a long cold winter is coming, so we are hardwired to pack on fat. Anyone can do it, and so did I. Here is how to operationally view the hypothalamus' relationship to weight gain.

In high school, I was a high jumper on the track team. As a senior, I was 6'2" tall and barely weighed 150 pounds. After graduating from high school, a friend and I bicycled from New Jersey to Florida, so I entered college the same weight. It was only after I stopped high jumping in college did I fill out with a bit more muscle and some fat, and was 165-170 pounds upon graduation. Today I weigh 170-175 pounds at the time I am writing this chapter.

The most I have ever weighed was about 190 pounds, and that added weight was definitely more fat than muscle. From the perspective of my hypothalamus, which is unaware of the current abundant food supply, if a cold winter came along and food was scarce, I would have a much better chance of surviving if I weighed 190 pounds. Thus, my hypothalamus has "tasted" 190 pounds and is happy to get me up there again. And my hypothalamus has the added advantage at the moment because when I write, I tend to become obsessed with writing and I exercise less. This means I must be very "mindful" about what I am putting in my mouth and how often I eat when I am in heavy writing mode.

How the body defends added fat mass – the body weight set point
Whatever body weight we achieve, it is recognized by the brain as a new and "proper weight for survival," about to which body metabolism is "set"; thus, the term body weight set point. I wish this were not true; however, research clearly indicates that body weight set points are modified to defend accumulated body weight and to promote the accumulation of additional weight gain.[3-9] You can easily think about this on a personal level. Either the scenario applies to you, a friend, or family member. And we have seen it happen to celebrities with weight problems. People will lose weight, then keep it off for a while, only to gain it all back and more. How does this happen? A recent weight loss study identified some of the potential mechanisms.

Thirty-four obese subjects completed a 62-week study to identify long-term hormonal responses to weight loss that might subsequently lead to rebound weight gain.[3] Hormonal assessments were performed at the beginning of the study, and at week 10 and week 62. The hunger promoting hormone ghrelin was measured, which was described earlier in Chapter 9 of this book. Multiple hunger-suppressing hormones were also measured in this study, including leptin, insulin, peptide YY, cholecystokinin, and amylin. Understanding the details about these hormones is not important for you; what is important is understanding that the body produces both hunger-promoting and hunger-suppressing hormones.

During the first 8 weeks, the Optifast very low calorie diet was used. This included the Optifast meal and two cups of low starch vegetables, which amounted to a total of 500 calories per day. This is basically a starvation diet. During weeks 9 and 10, low-glycemic whole foods were introduced, meaning that the subjects were acclimated to a diet that was low in refined sugar and flour. They were also educated about maintaining long-term dietary changes and exercise recommendations were provided. During weeks 11-62, dietary counseling and support involved bimonthly visits and telephone communications.

Not surprisingly, participants lost weight during the first 10 weeks, when they were closely monitored. They lost an average of 30 pounds within 10 weeks. Compared with baseline measurements, at weeks 10 and 62, the hunger-suppressing hormones were all reduced and there was an increase in hunger-promoting ghrelin. This would suggest that subjects would have been hungry during the entire study period, and this is exactly what they reported. However, they were not just "normal" hungry; they reported that their hunger and desire to eat was *elevated* during the entire study period. In everyday language, this of course means that they felt like they were starving.

As mentioned earlier, it is very difficult for us to resist the primitive drive of hunger, so all the subjects gave in and ate. At the end of the study, the average weight regain was 17 pounds. The authors concluded that, "there is an elevated body weight set point in obese persons and that efforts to reduce weight below this point are vigorously resisted."

What was lacking in this and other weight loss studies is a proper education about weight gain. Study participants are never educated in the fashion outlined in the many "why we are fat" chapters in this book. People who are overweight do not understand that we *all* have an instinctual drive to overeat, which is augmented by stress, sleep loss, and an inflamed hypothalamus. Weight loss study participants and people in the general population are mislead into thinking they should eat less food, when in fact, they should "overeat" low calorie anti-inflammatory foods so they feel full. People also need to understand the nature of the body weight set point and how to exert control over it, which you can do.

Accepting that we have a body weight set point

Practically speaking, we should understand that every one of us has a body weight set point that is vigorously defended – this means that your body will resist your efforts to lose weight even if your body and brain are *not* inflamed. The problem is magnified for overweight and obese individuals because it is likely they have the added burden of chronic inflammation, which means their hypothalamus does not adequately turn off the sensation of hunger. Recall from above what I described as one of the most important statements in this book to understand for those who struggle with weight issues:

> Hypothalamic inflammation actually functions to *"increase the defended level of body weight."*[1]

In short, the goal of weight-related body physiology is to defend a high body weight because the stored calories can be used during times when food is scarce. This aspect of physiology applies to all of us. However, for overweight and obese individuals, there is an augmentation of this physiology. As described in the previous chapter, the hypothalamus is not able to turn off hunger sensations because chronic inflammation prevents the hypothalamus from responding to the hunger-suppressing actions of insulin and leptin.

What this means practically in our daily lives is that *you and I and everyone who reads or does not read this book, will spend our entire life battling the body weight set point system to varying degrees.* Winning the war against weight gain is absolutely achievable, so long as we understand the nature of the weight-gain battlefield as described in this book.

Knowing your weight gain enemy

The most efficient and perhaps the only way to defeat a sophisticated enemy or opponent, is to understand what one is up against. How difficult will the battle or upcoming competition be? This question drives opposing sports teams to study each other before they play. My impression is that most people fail to maintain normal weight because they have no idea about the weight gain physiology (a sophisticated enemy) that is stacked against them. Answer these three questions:

1. Did you know before reading the "why we are fat" chapters that if you are fat it is because the human body, for the purpose of survival, wants to be overweight?

2. Did you know that we are hardwired with an instinctual drive to overeat that is augmented by stress, a lack of sleep, and body inflammation?

3. Did you know that we all have body weight set points that must be negotiated and dealt with effectively?

Getting fat has little to do with one's genetic makeup, which is a common claim by those who struggle with weight gain. Getting fat is ultimately about a physiological mechanism related to survival that does not have utility in the modern age, which is then augmented by an inflammatory lifestyle.

Exercise can lower the body weight set point

Recall all of the benefits of exercise that were listed in Chapter 9 of this book:

- Generates an immediate reward/pleasure response
- Promotes a general feeling of well being
- Appetite suppressive effects
- Anti-depressive effects
- Anti-anxiety effects
- Anti-stress effects
- Anti-inflammatory effects

In addition to these benefits, a recent study identified that, "exercise directly influences the responsiveness of the central nervous system (CNS) circuits involved in energy homeostasis by allowing the defense of a lowered body weight."[8] Believe it or not, this is how scientists state that exercise can definitely lower your body weight set point. This is very good news for us. We can reset our body weight set point with exercise so there is less of a vigorous biological drive to regain weight after weight loss.

Eating to lower the body weight set point
There is no scientific evidence that I am aware of that conclusively demonstrates how diet alone can lower the body weight set point. My impression is that there is no such relationship based on the physiology that I have studied. Do not worry though; this is fortunately not a weight loss deal-killer. All you have to do is eat anti-inflammatory foods until you are full and no longer hungry AND then be *respectful* of these feelings. It is impossible for a body to put on extra fat if it is fed large amounts of anti-inflammatory vegetation.

What to do on a daily basis
With all the societal and psychological issues that we must contend with that add to the stress and confusion of life, we need a simple mental plan to maintain proper weight. My suggestion is to create positive self-talk that will become your normal mindset for dealing with dietary and body weight issues. Here is a list of ten statements that you can use to train yourself to effectively manage your weight on a daily basis:

1. I accept that fat gain is a biological drive based on primordial survival issues. Fat gain is not my personal shortcoming or something unique to me and my genetic makeup. It is a human condition and anyone can get fat.
2. I will stop eating when my gut feels full, even if my brain lies to me and says I am still hungry.
3. I understand that my feeling of hunger, even though I am full, is an illusion created by my inflamed hypothalamus, which will go away in the very near future.
4. When I am full and cannot help myself but to eat more, I will only eat vegetables or fruit.
5. If I screw up and eat inflammatory foods, I will just accept that the primordial survival mechanism, stress, or a lack of sleep momentarily got the best of me. I will not flog myself and dive deep into despair about my failing and further punish myself with ice cream, cookies, donuts, chips, etc.
6. I will identify my stressors and get rid of every stressor I can.
7. I will get at least 6 hours of sleep per 24-hr day/night cycle.
8. I will exercise every day to feel better, reduce stress, inhibit my appetite, and reset my body weight set point to a healthy, normal level.
9. I will remove from my home every ounce of food that is pro-inflammatory. Only anti-inflammatory foods will enter my home.
10. I will accept that I am, like almost everyone else on earth, a dietary crackhead and treat myself accordingly.

Repeating or reading these every day is useful. This is how advertising works; repetitive stimulation, which eventually motivates us to buy whatever is being sold. Our brains need to be *sold* on these ten statements related to eating and body weight so that we can achieve and remain a healthy weight.

Obviously, #10 on the list is a new concept, unless you have read *The DeFlame Diet* book and/or some of my articles. While I have discussed dietary crack previously in this book, this is the first chapter wherein I suggest that we accept that we are dietary crackheads. Unfortunately, it is true that our human brains evoke an addiction-like response when we eat refined carbohydrates. And since white sugar and flour looks very similar to crack cocaine, it makes good sense to refer to these calorie sources as *dietary crack*. And because we desire these foods and have an addiction response to them, this makes us "dietary crackheads," in my opinion. This topic will be the focus of the next two chapters.

References

1. Wisse BE, Schwartz MW. Does hypothalamic inflammation cause obesity? Cell Metab. 2009;10:241–2.
2. Stoger R. The thrifty epigenotype: an acquired and heritable predisposition for obesity and diabetes? BioEssays. 2008;30:156–66.
3. Sumithran P, Prendergast LA, Delbridge E, et al. Long-term persistence of hormonal adaptions to weight loss. N Engl J Med. 2011;365:1597–604.
4. Harris RB. Role of set-point theory in regulation of body weight. FASEB J. 1990;4:3310–8.
5. Keesey RE, HirvonenMD. Body weight set-points: determination and adjustment. J Nutr. 1997;127:1787S–83S.
6. Levin BE, Keesey RE. Defense of differing body weight set points in diet-induced obese and resistant rats. Am J Physiol. 1998;274:R412–9.
7. Dokken BB, Tsao TS. The physiology of body weight regulation: are we too efficient for our own good? Diabetes Spectrum. 2007;20:166–70.
8. Krawczewski Carhuatanta KA, Demuro G, Tschop MH, Pfluger PT, Benoit SC, Obici S. Voluntary exercise improves high-fat diet induced leptin resistance independent of adiposity. Endocrinology. 2011;152(7):2655–64.
9. Briggs DI, Lockie SH, Wu Q, Lemus MB, Stark R, Andrews ZB. Calorie-restricted weight loss reverses high-fat diet induced ghrelin resistance, which contributes to rebound weight gain in a ghrelin-dependent manner. Endocrinology. 2013;154:709–17.

Chapter 14
Why we are fat – we are all dietary crackheads

The reason for designating sugar/flour products as dietary crack is because they are white powders and once we get a taste for them, most of us crave them for our entire lives and this is certainly the case for me. This is the same response that people have when they take crack cocaine just one time. The obvious difference is that crack cocaine kills people quickly, whereas dietary crack leads to the development of chronic inflammatory diseases like cancer, heart disease, Alzheimer's disease, etc., which kill us slowly over time.

Consider the power of dietary crack as demonstrated during a first exposure event in a child. Several parents have relayed a similar story to me. The parents of a 2-year old told me that they never let their child eat any dietary crack until their second birthday, when they allowed a piece of birthday cake to be eaten. This led to a profound reward/pleasure response. The child lifted pieces of cake upwards toward the sky with outstretched arms while making sounds of happiness and pleasure. This does not happen when you give a child broccoli or eggs or fish, or other whole foods…this only happens with dietary crack. Each parent told me that they were truly amazed by their child's excessive emotional reaction to dietary crack.

In my own experience, I remember as a kid asking my mother, "Mom, what's for dessert?" Why did I (and mostly likely you) ask this question? We asked because we developed a taste for the combination of sugar and flour at an early age because desserts taste really good.

What does "taste really good" mean from a neurobiological and neurobehavioral perspective? It means that we feel good, and *we all like to feel good* as often as we can; it is hard-wired into our nervous systems to pursue pleasure and avoid pain, which is very similar to the "happiness" issue discussed earlier in Chapter 2. Neurologically and emotionally, our brain registers a *pleasure* response from eating desserts, and for most of us, our first experience with the "dessert-induced pleasure response" was before the age of three or four. In other words, long before we are old enough to have adequate cognitive skills to understand the biochemical nature of desserts and the related pleasure response, we had a "reward" or addiction experience. We equated the "good" taste as being "good" food and we have desired it ever since. It is really that simple, which is why most people suffer emotionally when they consider giving up dietary crack.

From a psychological and neurobiological perspective, the "good" taste represents a temporary "state of happiness." As described earlier in Chapter 9, stress-induced eating has been studied from a metabolic perspective and is known to be associated with the increased consumption of comfort foods, such as desserts. This is because a temporary altered state of pleasure is generated when we eat dietary crack, which takes our focus away from stressful or unhappy situations. This is the same reason people abuse alcohol and drugs. Researchers who study addiction refer to a pleasurable response as "reward."

There are special sectors of our brains referred to as the "reward pathway." Specifically, it is often called the mesolimbic dopamine reward pathway and can also be called the mesolimbic system. Anything that gives us pleasure/reward activates this pathway - even exercise. So it is important to generate reward from healthy lifestyle choices.

In the case of drugs, when the "high" wears off, the abuser wants more drugs to get back into the reward state. In the case of food abuse, the state of pleasure lasts only as long as the taste buds are activated, which helps to explain why people overeat comfort foods. Consider the following fact: when most of us get close to finishing a dessert or anything that tastes good (reward), we get a bit of sad feeling because we know the pleasure/reward will soon end. We then start thinking about the next time we can get a taste of "dietary crack," or instead just have some more at that moment.

Researchers have actually demonstrated that brain reward centers become active when we merely look at dietary crack. This is because the reward centers "turn on" due to the anticipation of eating dietary crack. This occurs with everyone, whether one is thin, fat, or in between. However, if you are overweight or obese, a greater number of reward regions in the brain become active[1], which means that overweight and obese individuals have to exert much greater efforts to stop themselves from consuming dietary crack. Clearly, the term "dietary crackhead" is really quite accurate.

At the end of 2013, many news outlets reported on research performed at Connecticut College on rats that demonstrated how eating Oreo cookies activated the same reward/addiction centers as cocaine and morphine. Just like most humans, the rats ate the cream-filled center first. The news outlets actually stated that researchers have shown that Oreos are more addictive than cocaine. This is very much overstating the findings and conclusions of the authors; however, what these and previous researchers have absolutely identified is that high sugar/fat foods stimulate the brains reward/pleasure centers in the same fashion as addictive drugs[1-5], which is thought to be why we eat them despite knowing they are bad for us. What you need to understand and never forget is that to both the human and rat brain, the sugar/flour/fat combination is "dietary crack."

It is not unreasonable to think that it is unfair that our brains are wired to be dietary crackheads. I would agree; however, this is the way it is and it is not going to change. So, we need to accept the fact that we humans are dietary crackheads, and we need to deal with it by going through our cabinets, refrigerator, and freezer right now and throwing away all dietary crack. Throw away every food that contains sugar, flour, refined grains, whole grains, omega-6 fatty acids, and trans fats. They stimulate addiction mechanisms and are pro-inflammatory. We need to be able to live life without dietary crack in our homes.

Dietary crackhead anatomy and physiology

I debated whether I should include this section about anatomy, and then considered that an accurate and non-complicated description would be helpful. Dietary crackhead anatomy and physiology involves the mesolimbic dopamine reward pathway as mentioned above. There are several anatomical areas of the brain that make up the limbic system, which is the area that controls all feelings and motivations to act.

The term mesolimbic refers to a specific component of the limbic system involving the dopamine reward pathway. The ventral tegmental area (VTA) in the upper brainstem called the midbrain is the brain region that produces dopamine. Neurons (nerve cells) start in the VTA and end in the nucleus accumbens (NA) of the limbic system (Figure 1). When the VTA is activated, its neurons release *dopamine* into the nucleus accumbens (NA), which leads us to pursue the "pleasure" or "reward" response that we would like to repeat as often as possible.

Figure 1

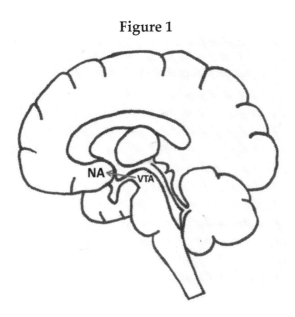

The VTA is not only activated by dietary crack, alcohol, and recreational drugs; multiple stimuli cause the VTA to release dopamine into the nucleus accumbens. In fact, anything that gives us pleasure does so by activating the dopamine system. Imagine anything you like and get pleasure from. The process first involves a sensation such as touch, sound, sight, or taste. This sensory input stimulates the VTA, which then stimulates the nucleus accumbens, which leads to reward/pleasure and the desire to keep doing whatever you find pleasurable. Even thinking about the things that give us pleasure activates the VTA-NA pathway to drive us to pursue reward.

So, a drug addict is really addicted to reward/pleasure response caused by the drug's ability to stimulate the VTA and nucleus accumbens. The reason why drug addicts and alcoholics relapse is because they seek the intense satisfaction they experience during the substance-VTA-nucleus accumbens-reward event, which is powerful and difficult to achieve without the addictive substance.

If one goes clean and gets off their addictive substance of choice, the chance for relapse is always present, which is why substance abusers avoid the environment that makes it easy to relapse. This is the same reason why staying off of dietary crack is so difficult. It is not because "diets don't work"; it is because the reward from dietary crack is so, so strong. That is, we love the feeling we associate with the taste of dietary crack. It is also very difficult to avoid these foods whenever we leave the home, which means temptation is everywhere.

This is why it is important for the 2/3s of the population that is overweight to understand that now and forever more they are and will be devoted dietary crackheads. Thus, they must create an environment and daily schedule that does not facilitate the exposure to, and consumption of, dietary crack.

A final point to never forget about the dietary crackhead

My brother Tom (on the cover of this book) did not eat a lot of desserts, soda, and candy (sugar/flour calories) to become obese. As described in the introduction, he overate chips, dips, deli sandwiches, deep fried foods, cheese, bread, pizza, and pasta. He is one of the rare people who does not have a sweet tooth, which is very helpful for proper weight management. In contrast to Tom, the vast majority of people cannot get enough sugar/flour calories. A mouse study appears to have revealed a potential reason for our obsession with sugar/flour calories.[1]

Mice, like humans, have a preference for sugar. They choose to drink sugared water when given the opportunity, just like humans. Scientists identified that taste receptors are not required for mice to develop a strong preference for sugared water. They utilized mice that were engineered to not have sweet receptors on their tongue. These mice that did not have sweet receptors, so they could not taste the sugar, still developed a strong preference for the sugared water.[1] The exact reason for how this happens is not understood; however, it may be that we get a reward response from calories independent of flavor.[6,7] No matter the mechanism, this finding demonstrates the power that sugar has over our nervous and behavioral systems - it appears that animals and humans are all dietary crackheads. In short, we are no match for the power of sugar, which is why you should keep desserts, pastries, soda, candy, etc., out of your home.

References
1. Lutter M, Nestler EJ. Homeostatic and hedonic signals interact in the regulation of food intake. J Nutr. 2009;139:629-32.
2. Gearhardt AN et al. Can food be addictive: public health and policy implications. Addiction. 2011;106:1208-12.
3. Gearhardt AN et al. Neural correlates of food addiction. Arch Gen Psych. 2011;68:808-16.
4. Lennerz BS et al. Effects of dietary glycemic index on brain regions related to reward and craving in men. Am J Clin Nutr. 2013;98:641-47.
5. Winter SR et al. Elevated reward response to receipt of palatable food predicts future weight variability in healthy-weight adolescents. Am J Clin Nutr. 2017;105:781-89.

6. de Araujo IE et al. Food reward in the absence of taste receptor signaling. Neuron. 2008;57:930-41.

7. de Araujo IE. Circuit organization of sugar reinforcement. Physiol Behav. 2016;164(Pt B):473-77.

Chapter 15
How to deal with our dietary crackhead

I am 58 years old as I finish this book and I currently weigh about 170 pounds, which is about what I weighed when I was a senior in college. I did weigh as much as 190 pounds in my late 30s, but lost the 20 pounds of fat and have kept it off ever since. The only way I am able to do this is to override the desires of the dietary crackhead and force myself to exercise, keep dietary crack out of my home, and almost never eat dietary crack in restaurants and coffee shops. Even by doing this, I can still overeat high-calorie, healthy anti-inflammatory foods, such as nuts or heavy cream on frozen cherries or blueberries. When I do this, I can easily gain 2-5 pounds, so I have to battle against the eating beast of the mesolimbic system and force my will over the various drives to overeat. The only way for us to do this is to actively engage our prefrontal cortex of the brain.

In this chapter, the picture of the brain (Figure 1 on the next page) also shows the prefrontal cortex. This is the part of your brain that observes and thinks about the reward/pleasure drives that are taking place in the nucleus accumbens.[1-3] The prefrontal cortex is also the region of the brain wherein thinking and reasoning occurs. It is the prefrontal cortex in the brain region that can go through a thinking process about how often you should engage in reward and if it is good for you. In contrast, the mesolimbic VTA-nucleus accumbens pathway is ALWAYS functioning to motivate us and drive us to engage in all manners of reward behaviors. From a scientific perspective, it is more accurate to describe the mesolimbic pathway as the desire and motivation pathway that drives us to realize reward and is not the pathway that experiences pleasure itself – however, for the purpose of this book, this differentiation does not really matter as this is not a neuroscience book.

Figure 1

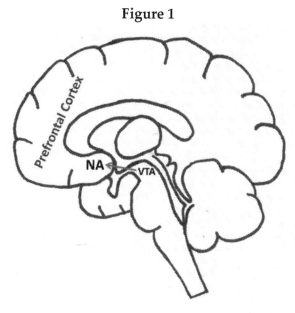

The prefrontal cortex is the only part of the brain that can send inhibitory signals to the reward pathway to override the drive to engage in reward activities like eating dietary crack. This means that we have to use the prefrontal cortex to override the constant motivation created by the mesolimbic system to abuse dietary crack – every day we must exercise to burn calories, keep dietary crack out of the home, and avoid dietary crack environments throughout the day. If you do not do this, you will gain weight; it is mostly unavoidable.

If you do not "wake up" your prefrontal cortex to the realization that the mesolimbic system will always motivate you to eat dietary crack, it is easy for the mesolimbic system to "take over" the conversation in the brain and utilize the prefrontal cortex to justify the avoidance of exercise and the ongoing consumption of dietary crack. This is called *rationalizing*. The prefrontal cortex can rationalize why it is okay to follow the lead of the mesolimbic reward system. We can even use the prefrontal cortex to rationalize why it is okay to let the mesolimbic system completely run our lives, which leads to overeating and other inappropriate behaviors, such as infidelity, spousal abuse, bullying, predatory business behaviors, lying, cheating, etc., because of the sick "pleasure/reward" it can generate for some. This is because it is the prefrontal cortex that "thinks" about how great the pleasure was and rationalizes why the activity should be repeated again and again and again.

So, the goal should be to psychologically and/or spiritually "live" in the prefrontal cortex, which has also been called the "seat of reason." In other words, *we* must "sit" in the "seat of reason" for the purpose of making proper life choices in general, and for the purpose of this book, avoiding dietary crack. Operationally, it is important to understand that none of us naturally sits in the "seat of reason"; we must, depending on your view of life, psychologically and/or spiritually place ourselves there by choice, as an active effort. With this in mind, lots of things can prevent us from sitting in the seat of reason and also kick us out of the seat, which causes us to live in the mesolimbic system often without evening knowing it. Three of the more powerful forces that prevent us from psychologically/spiritually sitting in the seat of reason are stress, lack of sleep, and lack of exercise, each of which was described in previous chapters.

So, what should you do? You must act like a parent disciplining a child's mesolimbic system; only in this case *it is your own mesolimbic system that you must discipline.* And you must realize that your mesolimbic system is no different from that of an infant or child. The mesolimbic system never matures; its only function is pleasure/reward from sensory stimuli such as dietary crack. This same approach for dealing with food choices and weight control also applies to the impulse control and self-regulation needed for dealing with other temptations - drugs, alcohol, sex, and gambling being the most problematic.

Who is manipulating your mesolimbic system?

Advertisers are quite aware of mesolimbic physiology, which is why product advertising is designed to link a product with a reward/pleasure experience. Advertising efforts entice you to imagine how good you will feel if you buy this new car, television, stereo system, gadget, etc. In other words, advertisements directly appeal to the mesolimbic dopamine reward pathway.

Consider the television commercials you watch that promote various foods. Have you ever watched a commercial that promotes the purchase and consumption of Brussels sprouts and kale? Neither of these vegetables induces a pleasure response that compares to the pleasure response induced by inflammatory foods such as desserts, pizza, French fries, onion rings, soda, or fast food hamburgers. Interestingly, the cost of manufacturing inflammatory foods is inexpensive, which allows for substantial advertising dollars to be invested in the activation of our mesolimbic dopamine reward system.

We need to understand that the consumption of foods made of sugar, flour, grains, trans fats, and omega-6 oils is good for food manufacturers, which I refer to as the food industrial complex, but not good for us. These foods are cheap so profits are large. On the consumer side of the equation, these foods are pro-inflammatory and lead to disease, which leads to a dependence on medications, which is good for drug manufacturers, which I refer to as the pharmaceutical industrial complex, but not good for us. Now consider the commercials for various medications...they manipulate the mesolimbic system by linking feeling good, or reward, with taking a medication. And since everyone wants to feel good, drug sales increase year after year. It is a multibillion dollar industry.

Without knowing it, we are all, to varying degrees, "mesolimbic victims" of the advertising that we let into our brains that lead to the predictable primitive behavioral response of pleasure pursuit that is expected by the advertisers. In order to DeFlame your body, you must reclaim your brain – in other words, you must reclaim, or claim for the first time, dominion over your mesolimbic dopamine reward system.

How to manage the manipulation of your mesolimbic system
<u>Identify and get to know your mesolimbic system</u>
Sit in a room without any sensory distractions – this is best to do at night or very early in the morning when the world is quiet. Now it is just you and your brain without any external sensory distractions.

Think about something that you like very, very much. It can be healthy or unhealthy; it does not matter what it is, and it does not need to be about food. Notice how the thing/activity you especially love makes you feel good – you are having a reward experience. If you really concentrate on your likes, you may feel the motivation to go and experience reward/pleasure for real. This will happen for me if I think about surfing or playing golf or landscaping my yard. As I write this paragraph and think about these things, I want to go do them right now, but I can't because I need to finish this chapter. So, I have to use my prefrontal cortex to deny the desires of my mesolimbic system.

Now think about the last time you ate pro-inflammatory foods (dietary crack). You had a choice to engage your prefrontal cortex and stop yourself. Unless you had completely mindlessly given into the mesolimbic system, in which there would have been no prefrontal cortex activity at all, you probably considered for a few seconds about making the choice to go ahead and eat the dietary crack. In other words, if we did not have a prefrontal cortex there would be no moments of consideration, and we would gobble up everything in sight. You need to work on capturing those moments of consideration and make them very conscious. This will help you occupy the "seat of reason" so you are very present in the moment; for in that moment you can use the prefrontal cortex to inhibit the mesolimbic pathway. Whenever you have the opportunity, I suggest that you practice engaging the prefrontal cortex. This is easy to do since temptation stimuli is everywhere around us...all one needs do is turn on the television. Or you can go to a restaurant and have a practice session.

In more common language, what I have described above is similar to the concept of delaying gratification. The mesolimbic system is the gratification system. In the context of weight loss and weight management, it is more about controlling gratification, rather than delaying it. To lose body fat, achieve normal weight, and then maintain a proper body weight, you will need to control gratification for the remainder of your life. This should not be viewed in the negative sense at all – it will allow you to have a much more healthy and vibrant life, so "controlling gratification" should be embraced wholeheartedly.

Do not deliver unhealthy ammunition to the mesolimbic system
Since most of us are fairly weak-willed when it comes to dietary crack, a key behavioral technique is to never buy it when you shop for groceries. Only anti-inflammatory foods should enter your home. Instead, if you have to eat dietary crack, reserve one day a week for it and make sure you buy only one serving if you bring it into your home. Otherwise, make the process of eating dietary crack something you do outside your home, and again, only one day a week. Keep your home pure and free of pro-inflammatory foods.

So far, I have only described the mesolimbic system in a fashion that may be perceived as negative; as if humans would be better off without a mesolimbic system. This is not at all the case. We need the mesolimbic system, for without it we would never feel pleasure/reward or drive to achieve any goal. The key is to train the mesolimbic system to experience reward/pleasure from activities that are beneficial for ourselves and others.

Retrain your mesolimbic pathway to support health
Direct your mind to behave as if you are in training for an athletic event or to look good for a physique contest, high school reunion, wedding, beauty show, going to the beach, or whatever you want, so long as it requires you to look and feel your best. People engaged in such physical training are focused on their goals and especially on how great they will feel when they achieve their

goals, which is the secret to sticking to any training program - a positive mesolimbic outcome. This makes eating anti-inflammatory foods and exercising daily an easy program to stick with and it is a way to purposefully engage the mesolimbic system in a healthy manner.

It is very important to understand that the human brain does very well when it is directed to achieve defined goals. For this reason, all self-help books implore us to work on our goals. Perhaps the most famous book of all is *Think and Grow Rich* by Napolean Hill, which is a very worthwhile text to read and re-read. The key point to understand about goals is that a goal-oriented mind is much more focused and less distracted by mesolimbic temptations.

<u>Exercise regularly to support healthy mesolimbic function</u>
Exercise has been described previously as having many benefits. They are listed here again:

- Generates an immediate reward/pleasure response
- Promotes a general feeling of well being
- Appetite suppressive effects
- Anti-depressive effects
- Anti-anxiety effects
- Anti-stress effects
- Anti-inflammatory effects
- Resets body weight set point lower

These are universal benefits of exercise for those who regularly exercise. It takes about a week to a month for non-exercisers to start to enjoy these benefits. If you are a non-exerciser, you now understand the timeframe you may be dealing with before the benefits kick in. It is especially important to ease into exercise if you have been a committed couch potato.

Notice that all the beneficial responses of exercise significantly outweigh the momentary pleasure derived from eating dietary crack. It is very important to never view exercise as only a means to burn calories. Exercise also generates a reward/pleasure response and reduces many of the promoters of weight gain including depression, anxiety, stress, and an elevated body weight set point.

It should be obvious that exercise is extremely important. You need to work with your exercise intensity and identify what is best for you to facilitate effective mesolimbic management.

Humor and mesolimbic reward
Several studies have identified that humor activates the mesolimbic reward centers.[4,5] This means we need to laugh and have fun.

The first time I ever caught a wave on my stand up paddleboard, when the ride ended I started laughing. It was so much fun that I laughed and laughed. It was a totally awesomely positive mesolimbic event; which happens many times when I surf. In this case, I was able to get the combined benefits of great exercise with laughter and joy. I do not surf as much as I used to so this is no longer a regular experience for me. However, I can think about it and still generate a pleasure state in my mind.

The point of describing my surfing experience is to demonstrate that you have many options for generating laughter, fun, and joy. You can always go right to the internet and watch some videos of your favorite comedian.

Never giving up
The main thing that you should keep in mind is to never give up and to not lose hope. Most people fall prey to dietary temptation and if you do, do not beat yourself up about it. Just "wake up" your prefrontal cortex and get yourself back into the "seat of reason." When we humans commit ourselves to achieving a goal, the outcomes are sometimes remarkable.

References
1. Noel X et al. The neurocognitive mechanisms of decision-making, impulse

control, and loss of willpower to resist drugs. Psychiatry. 2006;3(5):30-41.

2. Knoch D, Fehr E. Resisting the power of temptations: the right prefrontal cortex and self-control. Ann NY Acad Sci. 2007;1104:123-134.

3. Mendez MF. The neurobiology of moral behavior: review and neuropsychiatric implications. CNS Spectr. 2009;14:608-20.

4. Mobbs D, Greicius MD, Abdel-Azim E, Menon V, Reiss AL. Humor modulates the mesolimbic reward centers. Neuron. 2003;40(5):1041-8.

5. Franklin RG Jr, Adams RB Jr. The reward of a good joke: neural correlates of viewing dynamic displays of stand-up comedy. Cogn Affect Behav Neurosci. 2011;11(4):508-15.

Chapter 16

Why we are fat – we have the wrong bacteria in the gut

To really understand gut bacteria, one really needs a degree in microbiology. This is because the relationship between the human body and its resident population of bacteria is highly complex. On a basic level, it is important to understand this fact: eating sugar, flour, and refined oils, which make up almost 60% of calories consumed by Americans, will cause a shift in the gut bacteria population that promotes inflammation and weight gain. This fact should be considered with this additional information in mind:

> For many years, it was believed that the main function of the large intestine was the reabsorption of water and salt and the disposal of waste (feces). However, this view was far from complete, as it did not consider the activity of the microbial content of the large intestine. It is now clear that the complex microbial ecosystem in our intestines should be considered as a separate organ within the body, with a metabolic capacity that exceeds the liver by a factor of 100.[1]

This means that what we feed our gut bacteria can have a massive effect on body metabolism and push us toward health if we eat properly, or disease if we flame up on pro-inflammatory foods.

It is actually quite difficult to comprehend the amount of bacteria living in the human body. This is because bacterial cells vastly outnumber human body cells. In fact, bacteria are so densely populated in the human colon that even after one does the preparatory work for a colonoscopy and the colonic walls are visible when viewed through the colonoscope, the colon is still teaming with bacteria because they are super tiny and everywhere. In short, there are more bacteria in our digestive system than there are cells in our body. Another example of the vastness of bacteria in our colon is the not well-known fact that at least half the mass of a bowel movement is made of bacteria.

On earth there are over 50 different phyla, or groups, of bacteria; however, the human-associated bacteria belong to four, those being Firmicutes, Bacteroidetes, Actinobacteria, and Proteobacteria. The Firmicutes and Bacteroidetes groups account for more than 90% of all the bacteria in the human colon.[2] There is normally a balance between these two dominant groups of bacteria; however, this balance can shift and lead to weight gain.

When researchers compared the bacterial balance between lean and obese individuals, it was determined that obese individuals have larger amounts of Firmicutes. The problem with an overabundance of Firmicutes is that these bacteria are very efficient at extracting extra calories from food, which is then absorbed from the digestive tract into body circulation and adds to body fat mass.[2] I have heard overweight people say that all they have to do is look at bread, pasta, or desserts and they gain weight, which is of course impossible and quite the exaggeration. However, there is an element of truth to this statement. A Firmicutes-dominated bacterial population will allow for greater calorie absorption from a given food compared to lean people with a normal bacterial population.

Not surprisingly, sugar and flour cause a "bloom" or overgrowth of Firmicutes and a reduction in anti-inflammatory bifidobacteria[3] In other words, sugar and flour, which represent about 40% of total calories in the average American's diet, serve to "feed" the overgrowth of the specific group of bacteria (Firmicutes) that promote weight gain.

So, the obvious solution to the Firmicutes overgrowth and related weight gain problem is to avoid sugar and flour. If we do this, we will naturally have to eat more vegetables and fruit, which not only have less calories that facilitate body weight reduction, but are also rich in needed vitamins and minerals. Additionally, vegetables and fruit have unique substances called polyphenols that support proper body weight.

Polyphenols are the colorful pigments found in vegetables and fruit. It is well known that polyphenols are not highly absorbed by the digestive tract. This means that polyphenols travel through and DeFlame the small and large intestines. It turns out that polyphenols function to inhibit the overgrowth of Firmicutes and thus, help to maintain the proper balance between Firmicutes and Bacteriodetes.[4] Clearly, we should all be consuming liberal amounts of colorful vegetation, which is especially important for those wishing to lose body weight - they are highly nutritious, low in calories, and help to create a weight loss profile of gut bacteria. For more inflammation about polyphenols, see Chapter 24 in *The DeFlame Diet* book.

References
1. Possemiers S et al. The intestinal microbiome: a separate organ inside the body with the metabolic potential to influence the bioactivity of botanicals. Fitoterapia. 2011;82:53-66.
2. DiBaise JK, Zhang H, Crowell MD et al. Gut microbiota and its possible relationship with obesity. Mayo Clin Proc. 2008;83(4):460-69.
3. Sandhu KV et al. Feeding the microbiota-gut-brain axis: diet, microbiome, and neuropsychiatry. Translational Res. 2017;179:223-44.
4. Rastmanesh R. High polyphenol, low probiotic diet for weight loss because of intestinal microbiota interaction. Chemico-Biological Inter. 2011;189:1-8.

Chapter 17

Why we are fat – the influence
of our sense of smell

When I was a kid my mother would shop at the local bakery for fresh rye bread, which means my young brain was exposed to the smell of fresh bread and all the other goodies. To this day, I can still remember how amazing it smelled in there. I can also remember how I felt internally motivated to eat all the baked goods in the shop. I have a similar olfaction (smell) memory of going to my grandmother's house for Thanksgiving. We walked into her house from the cold and were hit with the warm air that contained the delicious aroma of turkey, apple pie, and other holiday foods.

Most profound for me about these olfaction memories is that they are about 50 years old, which speaks to the power of smell in relation to the emotion of food "happiness" and the desire to eat everything in sight. It turns out that my experience is the norm, rather than the exception, which means that if you are reading this book, some version of the olfaction scenario I just described applies to you. In fact, scientists have studied the effect that smell has on our emotions and desire to eat.

First, it was discovered that odors, in general, evoke memories in a more profound fashion compared to visual or verbal cues.[1] Second, studies have demonstrated that cuing a person with very pleasant food odors, such as the smell of pizza or warm cookies can stimulate salivation, appetite, and consumption.[2] The same food odors can also increase food intake in particularly sensitive individuals, depending on their body mass index (BMI), level of dietary restraint, and reported impulsivity.[2]

Here is an example of how the information in this chapter plays out in real life. After my brother Tom (on the cover of this book) got off a plane and walked into the terminal, he happened to be in the right spot to watch an overweight guy catch a whiff coming from a Cinnabon bakery. The man stopped in his tracks, raised his head up, and turned his nose toward the smell. Without hesitating, he walked over and bought a cinnamon roll that contains 880 calories. In effect, the man, in that moment, was powerless against the pleasant food odor coming from Cinnabon, which caused him to consume 880 calories that he did not need.

If we are not careful and mindful of our emotional reactions to the smell of tasty food, we can easily end up in a moment of mindless overeating. Whenever I fly or go to a mall, I have to remind myself to be mindful and present in the moment, so as to not be swayed by all the smells that beckon me to eat. I suggest that you do the same.

Another consideration to keep in mind is the fact that the sense of smell is required for us to obtain normal, appropriate flavor from food when we eat it. People who lose their sense of smell complain that food tastes bland; it is without flavor.[3] In order to not lose weight, these people essentially have to force themselves to eat. The thought for us to keep in mind is that people who lose their sense of smell often lose weight[3], and this is because they are no longer controlled by the power of food pleasure/happiness. When we are confronted with pleasant food odors, we should understand that our desire to eat is often not hunger, but an olfactory induced craving for the food/pleasure happiness reward. We must be mindful of this and force ourselves to activate the prefrontal cortex to control our food-eating impulses so that we do not overeat.

References
1. Herz RS et al. Neuroimaging evidence for the emotional potency of odor-evoked memory. Neuropsychologia. 2004;42:371-78.
2. McCrickerd K, Forde CG. Sensory influences on food intake control: moving beyond palatability. Obesity Rev. 2016;17:18-29.
3. Henkin RI, Smith FR. Appetite and anosmia. Lancet. 1971;297:1352–53.

Chapter 18
Consumerism, obesity, and your health

The last several chapters described the many reasons why we get fat, which ultimately leads to chronic disease. Some try to perpetuate the notion that we are overweight and obese because we are affluent, which is not accurate. Many wealthy people are quite fit and very lean. Others attempt to perpetuate the notion that poorer people are obese because they cannot afford healthy food, which is also not true, as many poor people are lean and fit. They stay active and budget their money properly to buy healthy foods, which are readily available at discount stores such as Walmart and Aldi. In short, it is an absolute myth that one's income level has anything to do with fatness. We are obese because of the psychological, behavioral, addictive, and metabolic factors discussed in the last several chapters, and these various factors can be manipulated by marketers, which is precisely what appears to have happened.

I was born in 1960, so I am old enough to remember when it was the rare child or parent who was obese. When I was young, I had two great grandparents and all four grandparents, three of whom were born in the late 1800s. My great Aunt was born in 1913 and she lived to be almost 101. They all grew up in an era where virtually no one was obese.

If you compare the physical appearance of Americans in 1918 versus 2018, we look like two different nations. In 1918, Americans were hard-working people who saved their money, bought only what they needed, and ate far more whole foods. Sweets were the rare experience, save for an occasional dessert. Most people actually grew small to large portions of their food in their backyards. What has happened to America in the last 50-100 years?

In short, we have turned into a nation of consumers, which has been termed "consumerism." Compared to the early to mid-1900s, our manufacturing-based economy has virtually disappeared. You can go to YouTube and watch videos of Black Friday shopping – it is like a feeding frenzy during which people mindlessly buy mostly foreign-produced items they do not need with money they do not have. These videos epitomize our consumerist society. The transformation of America from a self-reliant manufacturing nation occurred during the same time that Americans became sedentary, mesmerized by television, and began to live on refined sugar, flour, and oils, which have been advertised to us in an ongoing basis.

Space does not permit a detailed description of the events that transformed America from a productive and prosperous nation into the world's most obese, over-sick, brain-numbed, and indebted nation, but it all happened in the last 100 plus years. If you have an interest in understanding the process, my recommendation is to watch a 4-part documentary available at topdocumentaryfilms.com called *The Century of the Self*. I mentioned this documentary in Chapter 2 of this book.

Briefly, *The Century of the Self* documents the life of Edward Bernays, the nephew of Sigmund Freud. He was a propagandist and was employed by the US government and top corporations during his lifetime. He even wrote a book called *Propaganda*.

One of the most powerful examples of Bernays' abilities to control public behavior involved cigarette smoking. Before 1929, women never smoked in public and hardly any smoked privately. This obviously meant that cigarette manufacturers were missing out on half of the adult population and they wanted to increase their revenue. Bernays was employed to figure out how to get women to smoke. He contacted a psychiatrist trained in Freud's psychoanalytic approach to find out what cigarette smoking means to women. In short, sexual and social issues were the dominant themes. Bernays contacted female socialites and invited them to walk in the New York City Easter Day Parade in 1929. At specified locations during the parade, the women lit up their "torches of freedom." After that, women began smoking all over America and Bernays' clients were very happy.

The depth of Bernays' influence over the last 100 plus years is shocking – he is a dominant figure in the emergence of our consumerist society. My suggestion again is to watch *The Century of the Self*. You will forever look at commercials and advertisements with a different mindset, which is very important in general and in the context of this book, from the perspective of weight management and disease prevention.

Next time you go into a coffee shop, notice the calorie sources in eyesight while you are waiting in line – they are all made of sugar, flour, and oils. Further consider that nearly all food industry commercials and advertisements are for non-whole food calorie sources that promote obesity. Our mesolimbic system is constantly being propagandized to indulge in foods to which the human nervous system's addiction circuitry is activated. Unless you are mindful of this, it is very difficult to muster up the will to resist. This means you have to exert dominion over your limbic system and *observe* how it is swayed by stress, lack of sleep, and sensory input (advertising propaganda) and then, *use your prefrontal cortex* to control your behavioral responses to make proper decisions.

Most people think that they are not controlled by propaganda and that is because "propaganda" is not advertised as "propaganda" that should be ignored. The best way to experience the degree to which we have been propagandized into being a devoted consumerist is to imagine being without certain things that we think we need. This can be clothing, toys, cars, furniture, social media, and dietary crack to name a handful.

Whenever I do presentations to doctors or layman and describe why we should avoid pro-inflammatory foods, particularly the sugar-flour-fat combination, several audience members observably suffer by verbally objecting or grimacing. They feel what I can best describe as separation anxiety when they imagine NEVER again eating French fries, donuts, pretzels, potato chips, bread, and similar nutrient-free refined calorie sources. If you experience suffering from this thought, then your mind has been taken over by dietary crack propaganda and dietary crack addiction issues. This anxiety/suffering response generated by a simple suggestion is likely due to the fact that almost no one spends time thinking about not eating these calorie sources that give pleasure.

Flaming dietary crack foods are all around us because they have been a firmly ingrained part of our culture for decades. We shop at the mall and go to the food court and flame up. We go to the movie theatre and get in line to pay extremely high prices for calorie sources to flame up with during the movie. We go to athletic events and flame up. We stand in line to check out at the supermarket and on shelves to the left and right is dietary crack at arm's length, tempting us to indulge. We go to get gas and all the stations now have stores that are packed full of dietary crack. We go to get a cup of coffee and our only option is dietary crack. We are constantly being propagandized to eat pro-inflammatory foods that almost all of us are addicted to.

Consider the fact that "mindless overeating by consumers" is a good business goal for the companies that sell low-nutrient pro-inflammatory calorie sources. The profit on these calorie sources is substantial compared to vegetables and fruit. Consider also how drug companies benefit from people overeating dietary crack. It insures that people will eventually be on one or multiple medications for life such as statins for cholesterol, metformin for blood sugar, anti-depressants, and anti-hypertensive drugs.

The television commercials for dietary crack and medications are impossible to avoid. I do not watch television at home and only do so when I am staying at a hotel. In December of 2014, I was at a seminar and was watching television on Friday night. In just one commercial break, I was exposed to multiple drug commercials in a row that included Tamiflu, Bayer Aspirin, Cialis, Ensure, and Chantix.

It can be bit depressing if you consider that most of us are manipulated by propaganda to buy pro-inflammatory foods and regularly use various medications. If you are bothered by this and wish you could do something to about it; we really only have one choice. We should recognize that we cannot stop the propaganda, so my suggestion is to not waste time trying to stop it. Our one option is to simply stop financially supporting the propagandists by embracing an anti-inflammatory lifestyle. By doing this, we will no longer funnel hard-earned money toward the consumption of pro-inflammatory foods and the directly related medical treatments that can be financially devastating. We should make it a goal to utilize medicine and surgery in only crisis situations; not as a lifestyle.

Chapter 19
Medical and workplace costs associated with obesity

Medical costs of obesity in 2008 dollars were estimated at $147 billion.[1] There are additional costs related to a loss of productivity in the work place - absenteeism related to obesity costs employers an estimated $3.38-6.39 billion per year.[1] All of the following diseases are more common in obese individuals[1]:

- All causes of death
- High blood pressure
- High LDL cholesterol, low HDL cholesterol, high triglycerides
- Type 2 diabetes
- Coronary heart disease
- Stroke
- Gall bladder disease
- Osteoarthritis
- Sleep apnea and breathing problems in general
- Some cancers (breast, endometrial, colon, kidney, gallbladder, liver)
- Low quality of life
- Mental illness such as depression, anxiety, and other mental disorders
- Body pain and difficulty with physical functioning

Obesity and its related diseases are completely non-discriminatory. People in every race and economic level suffer. Fortunately, wealth is not required to reverse obesity. We just need to stop overeating sugar, flour, and refined oils, and be more active. The solution is that simple, even though the process can be emotionally arduous as outlined in this book.

Societal benefits of proper weight management

Every several years, society goes through its upheavals. When you look at our sociopolitical environment now, it is clearly flamed up. This happens on a regular basis and is obvious if you look at it from the perspective of history. In my impression, sociopolitical emotions often go too far. The French Revolution is an obvious example of this that none of us lived through, which is why I am selecting it as an example that should not cause a reader of this book to become emotionally reactive. Too many heads rolled in France before calmer minds prevailed. Similar scenarios have happened in many countries.

In short, we are not properly taught about our emotions and how to control them to achieve the best benefit we can in a given situation, be it dietary, financial, social, or political. Believe it or not, dealing with the eating beast within is the best way to generally test your own emotional regulating ability. If we can control what goes into our mouths, we have a better chance of controlling our other behaviors, all of which are emotionally flavored.

The greater benefit of proper weight management is that it is good for society. Healthcare costs can be substantially controlled if we maintain normal body weight throughout life. Pursuing disease with poor lifestyle choices, as most people do, leads to the expression of lifestyle-induced diseases, which means less healthcare dollars for those who are unlucky to be stricken with disease or injury who, by no fault of their own, really need help.

References
1. CDC. Adult obesity causes and consequences.
   https://www.cdc.gov/obesity/adult/causes.html

Made in the USA
Columbia, SC
20 October 2018